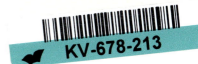

Pediatric Otorhinolaryngology

Advances in
Oto-Rhino-Laryngology

Vol. 23

Series Editor
C. R. PFALTZ, Basel

S. Karger · Basel · München · Paris · London · New York · Sydney

Pediatric Otorhinolaryngology

Volume Editor
B. Jazbi, Kansas City, Missouri

101 figures, 1 colour plate, and 16 tables, 1978

S. Karger · Basel · München · Paris · London · New York · Sydney

Advances in Oto-Rhino-Laryngology

Vol. 20: Otophysiology. International Symposium on Otophysiology. Eds.: J.E. HAWKINS, jr.; M. LAWRENCE, and W.P. WORK, Ann Arbor, Mich. VI + 542 p., 289 fig., 18 tab., 1973. ISBN 3-8055-1338-0

Vol. 21: Radiology in Oto-Rhino-Laryngology. Ed.: S. BRÜNNER, Copenhagen. VIII + 156 p., 69 fig., 23 tab., 1974. ISBN 3-8055-1632-0

Vol. 22: Audio-Vestibular System and Facial Nerve. Ed.: W.J. OOSTERVELD, Amsterdam. X + 220 p., 119 fig., 19 tab., 1977. ISBN 3-8055-2354-8

Cataloging in Publication
  Pediatric otorhinolaryngology / volume editor, B. Jazbi. – Basel, New York:
  Karger, 1978.
  (Advances in oto-rhino-laryngology; v. 23)
  1. Otorhinolaryngologic Diseases – in infancy & childhood I. Jazbi, Basharat,
  1932- ed. II. Title III. Series
  W1 AD701 v. 23 / WV 100 P371
  ISBN 3-8055-2674-1

© Copyright 1978 by S. Karger AG, 4011 Basel (Switzerland), Arnold-Böcklin-Strasse 25
Printed in Switzerland by Benziger AG, Graphischer Betrieb, Einsiedeln
ISBN 3-8055-2674-1

Contents

Preface

This volume has been prepared keeping in mind the paucity of adequate and up-to-date references on diagnosis and treatment of ear, nose and throat diseases in children. Because our concepts of management have been significantly altered in recent years by the tremendous advances in medicine in general and otorhinolaryngology in particular, I invited several colleagues who are well known for their interest, research and clinical expertise in pediatric otorhinolaryngology to share their experiences.

This issue on *Pediatric Otorhinolaryngology* is a result of teamwork. No single individual can claim total credit for it. I am very grateful for the generous response from all my friends and colleagues who, despite a multitude of other important commitments, agreed to contribute their work to this volume. The editorial task has been a rewarding experience as I have learned a great deal from all of them.

My sincere thanks to Ms. GREDER and the staff of S. Karger AG for their help and understanding, as no book of this scope goes to press without extensive work and cooperation by the publishers.

BASHARAT JAZBI, M. D., D. L. O., F.A.A.P.
Professor and Chief – Otorhinolaryngology
University of Missouri, Kansas City, School of Medicine,
The Children's Mercy Hospital,
Kansas City, MO 64108 (USA)

Dedication

This volume of *Advances in Oto-Rhino-Laryngology* is dedicated to colleagues all over the world who are devoted to the teaching and practice of pediatric otorhinolaryngology.

BASHARAT JAZBI, M.D., D.L.O., F.A.A.P., Editor

Adv. Oto-Rhino-Laryng., vol. 23, pp. 1–21 (Karger, Basel 1978)

Secretory and Serous Otitis Media (SOM)

Jacob Sadé[1]

The Meir Hospital, Kfar-Saba, The Weizmann Institute, Rehovot, and
The Tel-Aviv University Medical School, Tel-Aviv

Introduction

Secretory otitis media is a common pathological entity, presenting a middle ear effusion behind an intact drum, without symptoms of acute infection. This effusion impedes the acoustic wave, resulting in most cases in some hearing loss. The physical character of the effusion varies, ranging from watery 'serous' to a rubbery-like 'secretory' effusion. Other synonyms are glue ear, catharal otitis media and tubotympanitis. The absence of overt inflammatory symptomatology and difficulties in clearing up the effusion have provided a basis for extensive speculations and confusion as to the nature and treatment of SOM. However, studies conducted over the last two decades have shed some light on the etiology of the disease and its effective treatment. Serous effusion is also seen in patients with carcinomas of the nasopharynx and after Barotrauma; however, these entities in all probability have a different pathogenecity and will not be discussed here.

The Clinical Picture

The main symptom of SOM is hearing loss – this is preceded by obvious URI or acute otitis media in some 65 % of cases. The hearing deficit is due to the presence of the effusion in the middle ear; however, the hearing loss is usually variable and unpredictable due to the variability in the quantity, physical character, and intratympanic topographic placement of the effusion [1].

---

[1] Established Investigator of the Chief Scientist's Bureau, Ministry of Health, Israel.

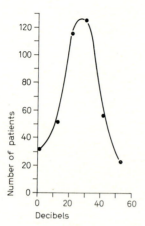

Fig.1. Hearing loss in 408 ears with SOM. Note the Gaussian distribution with an average of 28 dB.

Most affected by SOM are young children, constituting, hearing-wise, an 'uncomplaining population', and often below the age where audiometry is practical. This accounts for some difficulties in diagnosis; accordingly, this entity, which is the most common cause of hearing loss in children, is often not recognized [2, 3]. With time, SOM does clear up spontaneously in most cases; thus it is likely that the number of children and infants who have such an effusion at one time or another exceeds all conservative estimates.

Hearing loss is variable: Decibel-wise it has a Gausian distribution (fig. 1) – the average hearing loss is 28 dB [4, 5]. In the minority of cases (20%), it is only unilateral, in the rest it is bilateral. The hearing deficit is mostly noted by the mother or teacher – the child is rarely aware of it. It should be stressed that hearing loss has most probably a deleterious effect on a child's development only once it reaches a certain level. A bilateral 20-dB hearing loss or a unilateral 35-dB hearing loss will in all likelihood do little harm. It is because of this that the en masse treatment of the tremendous number of children 'afflicted' with SOM (about 5–10% of young school-children) should be regarded critically. On the other hand, once hearing loss has exceeded important levels and communication is jeopardized, proper treatment is mandatory.

Pressure and vertigo are only rarely associated with SOM and are present mostly in adults – some also may experience the sensation of liquid shifting place in the ear during head movements.

Pains is present only during, or immediately after, episodes of acute flare up – acute otitis media or upper respiratory disease do indeed frequently precede or appear as complications of SOM [6].

The Nature of the Middle Ear Effusion

A. Bacteriology

The effusion is often found to be sterile. However, bacteria can be cultured in 20–50 % of cases – these usually are the same found in acute otitis media [7, 8] (Haemophilos, Diplococci). Smears taken from many of the 'sterile' effusions do however show dead bacteria [8–10]. Though there has been speculation of a viral etiology, no evidence for this has been presented so far, which is hardly surprising in view of the very small percentage of acute otitis media yielding positive viral cultures [11]. It is interesting, however, to note that the incidence of SOM was reported to increase during viral epidemics [12].

The lack of bacteriological growth in cultures and the undramatic response to antibiotic therapy have served as a basis for much speculation in regard to the nature of SOM. The patient's previous history (infections) as well as a positive bacterial smears, the biochemical composition of the effusion and histopathological findings (see below) were ignored and 'allergic' or 'mechanistic' *(ex vacuo)* theories were advanced.

B. Cytology

Very large numbers of leukocytes are found in all effusions, many of which show engulfed dead bacteria [9]. Eosinophils, which were looked for extensively in an effort to link SOM with an allergic state [13] are, however, present only in very small numbers or completely absent [14].

C. Biochemistry, Rheology, and Physiology of Mucus

When a middle ear effusion is subjected to electrophoresis [15–17], one obtains a fraction which has no motility as well as a full spectrum of blood proteins. The non-motile fraction consists of a protein having sugar side-chains, it is PAS-positive and thus can be identified as a glycoprotein. The immotility of the glycoprotein is due to its being crosslinked into long polymer chains by S-S bonds. After splitting the S-S bonds, the fractions obtained can be separated electrophoretically and show some solubility. They consist of 'mucus monomers', indistinguishable from other mammalian 'mucus monomers', on the basis of their molecular weight (600,000 daltons) and amino acid and sugar compositions [18]. It is these molecules which give mucus its viscoelastic properties.

The viscoelastic properties of the effusion have a broad spectrum ranging from water (serous) to a semi-solid rubbery glue-like (secretory) material [19]. Efforts to *quantitate* these viscoelastic properties were so far rather fruitless due to the small quantities available from each sample. i.e. 0.1 to 0.3 ml per ear. Also, it is difficult to obtain samples of very viscous 'glue-like' effusions – the intermolecular forces binding the glycoprotein molecules are strong enough to prevent their 'separation'. Such a glue has in effect the properties of a 'semi-solid' rather than a fluid. This often results in great difficulties in removing the glue – even with a powerful suction. The rheological differences between effusions, i.e. their degree of viscoelasticity, is in effect not a function to the amount of water in them, as often assumed – it is actually a function of the amount of glycoproteins and the extent of them being crosslinked.

The middle ear lining – especially its anterior part and the Eustachian tube – are lined by a respiratory epithelium, which physiologically constitutes a muco-cilliary system [20, 21], and which secretes the mucus and is also responsible for its clearance. Speculation on clearance deficiency of the effusion, as the case in SOM is, as a result of its rheologic properties were natural.

Our experiments [22] have demonstrated that in effect mucus plays specific physiological role in such systems, i.e. it acts as an essential mechanical coupler to bring about effective transport by cilia (fig. 2): in depleted mucosas – which are devoid of mucus – no such transport took place. The coupler, in this case mucus, must have certain specific rheological properties – for example, its viscoelasticity must lie within a certain range – for transport to take place. One may speculate that both serous or excretory effusions cannot be cleared because they are out of the necessary range, i.e. either insufficiently or too viscoelastic [23].

On the basis of electrophoretic measurements, various γ-globulins [24–27], and enzymes [28–34], lysozyme [35] and prostoglandins [36] can be identified. These findings lead to speculation regarding the defensive and biological activities of the effusions. There is, however, so far no concrete evidence as to the actual operational (physiologic and pathophysiologic) significance of the various γ-globulins in the effusion. Thus, for example, MOGI et al. [37] have negated that the IgE levels found in SOM effusions have any particular significance when an atopic allergic factor is postulated. The

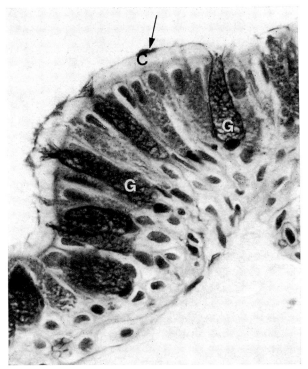

Fig. 2. Histological picture of a mucociliary (respiratory) epithelium. G = Mucus-producing cell (Goblet cell); C = cilia; arrow = mucus blanket. Note that the mucus blanket is emitted by the mucus cells and is deposited on top of the cilia.

various enzymes recovered from such effusions may well be simply evidence that cellular decomposition is taking place (of epithelial and white blood cells) – as in any other inflammatory exudate.

Summarizing: The middle ear effusion, which was considered for years to be a transudate of mysterious hydrostatic origin, is in effect a classic inflammatory exudate composed of dead epithelial cells, leukocytes, serum, dead or alive bacteria and mucus. The mucus gives the effusion its rheologic character. While there is a basis for speculation that these rheologic properties may be responsible for mucus clearance or non-clearance, this particular crucial question remains as yet open.

Diagnosis

While SOM as a clinical entity has been known for many years, its routine diagnosis is only relatively recent. Until about 20 years ago, only a few cases were recognized or treated. This might de due to greater awareness, to greater use of audiometry (a relatively new technique), and lately to the advent of tympanometry. It is also possible that there is a true increase in the incidence of SOM, possibly as a result of the routine treatment of acute otitis media with antibiotics, and the inconvenient paracentesis being practised less frequently. Antibiotic treatment might cause abatement in the symptoms of acute otitis media, but without the beneficial effects obtained when an abcessing ear is drained. This might result in retention of an effusion which is often sterile or has a small bacteria count. That such a course of events is also conductive to recurrent acute otitis media (i.e. an acute otitis media 'complicating' SOM) has been pointed out by Diamant [38].

Examination especially under magnification (fig. 3) of an ear drum with SOM will more often than not reveal signs of the effusion. Mostly a slight or conspicuously *bulging* drum is seen. Less often, fluid levels can actually be observed behind the drum; generally, however, the drum is opaque and has lost its semi-transparency, showing a certain vascular injection. When acute otitis media has recently preceded the examination, slight wet desquamation of the external epithelium covering the drum and the adjacent external canal can be noted.

Using the pneumatic otoscope, the drum is seen to move more slugishly than is normal – the notion that no movement is elicited when an effusion is present behind the drum – i.e. that the 'drum does not move' – is, however, incorrect.

With time, the drum may atrophy and two additional phenomena may occur. One is retraction, i.e. first stage of atelectasis, and the other is the appearance of granulation tissue at the posterior part of the anulus – the 'Herodion', described in detail elsewhere [39].

Audiometry shows *conductive* deafness – an average of 28 dB hearing loss [4, 5]. In a statistical sample of patients, there is actually a Gaussian distribution (fig. 1) in hearing loss.

In young children – and SOM is mostly seen in children – audiometry can be difficult or impractical due to the inability of the children to answer accurately whether they did or did not receive an acoustic stimulus. Here impedence measurements (tympanometry) are sometimes useful and this technique can be viewed as providing a practical objective way for diagnosing

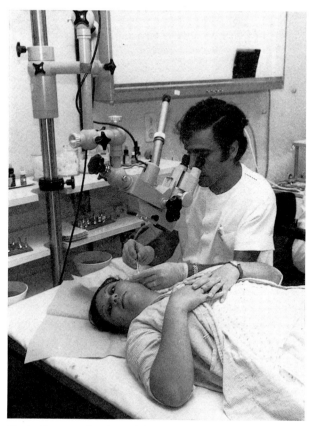

Fig.3. Ear examination with magnification, using the 'surgical' microscope and suctions (suction is on the right hand of the house officer who examines the patient).

SOM [40, 41]. A 'negative' value supposedly indicating middle ear negative pressure or 'flat curve' is recorded when an effusion is present in the middle ear. However, interpretation must be made with care. The information recorded is the effect of the effusion on the acoustic wave; *direct* intratympanic pressure measurements by BUCKINGHAM and FERRAR [42] and SADÉ *et al.* [41] have shown that often no negative pressure is to be found at all in SOM ears and, when there is, the average magnitude is only of the order of 5 mm H_2O.

Hearing loss due to SOM is usually dramatically improved immediately on introducing air into the affected ear. The air is introduced through the nose via the Eustachian tube with a Politzer bag, and provides evidence that the Eustachian tube is not 'blocked'. This is a valuable differential diagnostic test rather than a means of therapy, since improvement achieved this way is only temporary.

The Nose, the Adenoids and the Tonsils in SOM

In the past, the adenoids were considered as the main culprit in SOM and adenoidectomy (or even tonsillectomy) followed the finding of the typical effusion or suspicion of hearing loss in children. The sequence of events was seen thus: at first, adenoids obstructing the Eustachian tube. Subsequently, oxygen was supposed to be absorbed from the unaerated closed tympanic cavity – into the circulation, producing an intra-tympanic vacuum (fig. 4). This vacuum was postulated to provide the force to suction the transudate (the effusion) from the blood vessels into the tympanic cavity. Retraction of the ear drum was considered as supporting evidence, despite the fact that the tympanic membranes in the vast majority (over 90 %) of cases of middle ear effusion are either in their proper position or slightly bulging, rather than retracted. The viscous nature of most effusions was initially attributed to reabsorption of water from the effusions which were then supposed to become mucoid by concentration. This is in direct contradiction to the fact that no matter how much serum is concentrated, no mucoid substance is obtained. Interestingly, until about 15 years ago, there was total ignorance of the ability of the middle ear to produce mucus, or for that matter, that it had a mucociliary lining [16]. While there is some indication that adenoids are larger in SOM patients than in control groups, there is however so far no concrete evidence that they are pathogenetically involved in SOM. Although lateral nasopharyngeal X-rays may show the adenoids and the obstructed or unobstructed nasopharyngeal airway (fig. 5), quantitative measurement of the adenoid mass is difficult because of masking by the curve of the base of the skull and the height of the soft palate. Consequently, no reliable measurements of adenoids in SOM patients are so far available. Furthermore, convincing documentation that adenoidectomy (not to mention tonsillectomy) is beneficial, as far as the cure of SOM is concerned, has not been produced either. On the other hand, the percentage of SOM patients who have no 'enlarged' adenoids or have a recurrent effusion *after adenoidectomy* [43, 44] is astounding! 35 % and more claims that sinus infection or nasal pathology is more common in these children than in controls have also not been substantiated with data to date.

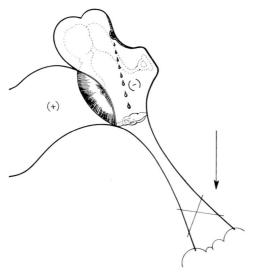

Fig.4. Schematic drawing of the popular 'ex vacuo' theory. Note tympanic cavity shows a hypothelical transudate from vascular origin due to a negative pressure. Arrow = Hypothelical obstruction of Eustachian tube by adenoids.

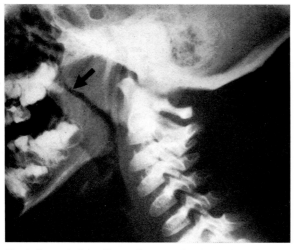

Fig.5. Lateral view of nasopharynx, showing enlarged adenoids (arrow) and narrow nasopharyngeal airway just below it.

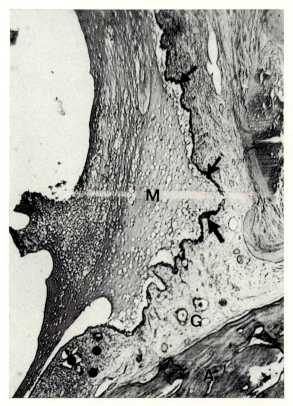

Fig.6. Histological section of middle ear with SOM. M = Inflammatory mucoexudate; arrows = metaplastic mucosa (PAS-positive), wherefrom the mucus originates; G = mucus glands in submucosa; A = bony framework of middle ear; three black dots = submucous thickly infiltrated with inflammatory cells.

Pathogenesis and Pathology

Histopathologic studies [45] of the middle ear lining of SOM patients show principally three phenomena: (1) an inflammatory process, i.e. inflammatory cells infiltrating the submucosa, edema and enlargement of capillaries; (2) a metaplastic process of the goblet cells, as seen in other inflammed mucosa, i.e. the number of goblet cells and actual glands has appreciably increased (fig.6, 7); (3) the Eustachian tube was found to be open throughout its whole length. In addition to this histopathological

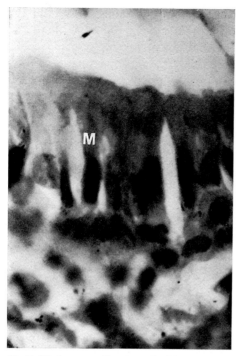

Fig. 7. Higher magnification of a histological section of the metaplastic middle ear mucosa (compare with fig. 2), showing all cells to have turned into mucus-synthesizing cells (M). In submucosa, numerous inflammatory cells are to be seen.

evidence, many patients (65 %) explicitly have a previous history of upper respiratory inflammatory disease. The effusion should be viewed therefore as a banal post-inflammatory exudate. Several questions now arise: (a) What is the origin of the exudate in those about 35 % of patients who do not have a history of inflammatory upper respiratory disease? (b) Why does the effusion promptly reappear in many ears after having been aspirated? (c) Why do a certain (albeit small) number of patients progress towards atelectatic ears? Is there an additional factor to inflammation?

There is evidence that a specific physiological condition, i.e. deficient aeration of the Eustachian tube, is that *additional* factor involved in SOM. It is the deficient Eustachian tube function which helps us understand those phenomena which an inflammatory process by itself cannot explain. While there is no evidence that Eustachian tube malfunction is related to an obstructive phenomenon, as has been postulated so often [46] (indeed, autopsies have revealed the tube to be actually wide open [45]), there is evidence that in these cases aeration of the middle ear is 'inadequate'. This is apparent from the beneficial surgical effect of ventilation of the ear, using a ventilating tube. Such ventilation causes prompt clearance of the effusion (whether the material is aspirated mechanically at surgery [41] or not! [41] and prevents its re-accumulation. On the other hand, HOLMQUIST and RENWALL [47] have also shown experimentally that SOM ears have a diminished ability to equilibrate artificially induced pressure. Also cleft palate patients, the majority of whom suffer also from SOM, have a congenital defect of the muscles governing the opening and the function of the Eustachian tube [48–50].

We do not know how much should be the rate of air flow via the Eustachian tube into a healthy ear, nor how much actually reaches the sick ear. Neither do we know the precise mechanisms which govern this process – though it is likely to be related to the muscles of the tube, which governs its opening. On the other hand, we do know that several inflammatory pathological entities are associated with 'under-aerated ears': accumulation and clearance deficiency of middle ear effusions, atelectasis, perforation of the drum (pars tensa), and last but not least, cholesteatoma. All of these conditions are associated with difficulties in equilibration of outside pressures, have an atelectatic tendency and are improved by surgical aeration with a ventilating tube. It is interesting to note that in most SOM cases these phenomena are likely to be transitory – 'once Eustachian tube malfunction does not necessarily mean always Eustachian tube malfunction'. Whether 'under aeration' of the middle ear be permanent or transitory, it is a factor to be considered from two viewpoints – pressure and gas composition.

A. Middle Ear Pressures

This popular and 'obvious' explanation leads to the concept that we are dealing with a middle ear underpressure phenomenon [51]. This explanation is based on the 'closed middle ear' model followed by gas absorption (mostly oxygen) and vacuum formation thereafter. In this assumption, we consider the venous (690 mm Hg) or capillary (720 mm Hg) pressures equilibrating with the atmospheric pressure (760 mm Hg). Thus, the differential (with capillary pressure, 760–720 mm Hg $= 40$ mm Hg, or 540 mm H_2O) would account for a vacuum of over 500 mm H_2O. Yet, when one measures directly the pressure in SOM ears, one finds an average negative pressure of about only 5 mm H_2O, a difference of two orders of magnitude [39, 41].

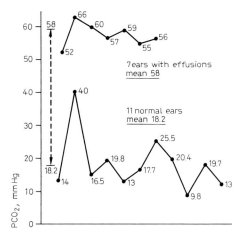

7ears with effusions
mean 58

11 normal ears
mean 18.2

Fig. 8. A comparison of CO_2 concentrations in normal ears (lower curve) with CO_2 concentrations found in SOM ears (upper curve).

B. Middle Ear Gas Composition

Once the air exchange rate falls in a closed system, a second factor should be taken into account, i.e. partial pressures of oxygen and carbon dioxide. Preliminary measurements (fig. 8) show a fourfold higher concentration of CO_2 in SOM than in the normal ear [52–54]. We have also provided both clinical and experimental tissue culture data which implicates such high CO_2 concentrations as affecting direction of cellular differentiation in general and, specifically, a shift in respiratory cell differentiation towards a cell population rich in mucus-producing cells [53–56].

Biopsy and autopsy material from SOM middle ear mucosa do indeed show impressive metaplastic shifts of the normal middle ear respiratory mucosa into strata of cell populations composed solely of mucus-synthesising cells [46, 57–60]. GUNDERSON and GLUCK [61] and later PALVA *et al.* [31] have reported that this situation reverses itself after ventilating tubes are introduced into the tympanic membrane.

Summarizing this chapter on middle ear aeration, it should be pointed out that it is known that the middle ear is not adequately aerated in various inflammatory middle ear disorders in general and in chronic SOM in particular. However, we do not have sufficient information to understand these phenomena adequately either qualitatively or quantitatively. This 'malfunction' can be considered either from the point of view of pressure – direct measurements show an *average* negative pressure of 2–5 mm H_2O in SOM cases – or from the point of view of gas composition where higher CO_2 concentrations than normal have been measured in SOM ears than in normal controls.

Natural History of SOM

With time and patience, the effusion will clear in most middle ears. The time factor is, however, quite meaningful as it is important whether hearing will return after 6 weeks – or 6 months or longer. In a certain number of cases, the effusion persists – even for years. Furthermore, in some cases progress is particularly slow and other parameters unrelated to the effusion itself but secondary to the combination of slow inflammation and middle ear under-aeration supervene; these are partial or total tympanic drum displacement towards the medial wall of the ear, i.e. atelectasis. Necrosis of the incus might also supervene, and there are reports of the development over time of central perforations [62] or even cholesteatomas (fig. 9) [7, 63].

Treatment

Treatment was originally routinely directed towards removal of the adenoids – they were viewed as obstructing the opening of the Eustachian tube. Later, transtympanic aspiration of the effusion was employed. At present, the thinking is that there is no certainty whether adenoidectomy is really beneficial [43, 44, 64] and, on the other hand, we know that in many cases the effusion will swiftly return after being aspirated.

However, aspirating the effusion from the middle ear restores hearing almost instantly to approximately normal, and restoration of hearing is our primary goal in SOM. To avoid reaccumulation of an inflammatory exudate (the 'glue' or effusion), a very small opening in the drum has to be kept open. This will ensure the 'proper aeration' of the middle ear for some time (as long as the ventilating tube will be functioning no mucus will reaccumulate in the middle ear and hearing will be good). In cases where this is indicated, a plastic micro-tube [64, 65] is inserted into the myringotomy incision to prevent its closure (fig. 10). The variety of such commercially available tubes is enormous; however, whatever tube is inserted at whatever place in the drum – the outcome is the same. After an *average* interval of about 6 months, all tubes are rejected. The mechanism through which this happens is two-

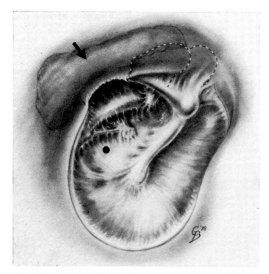

Fig. 9. Drawing of an atelectatic drum grade 3 (black dot). Below the atelectasis, the stapes is to be seen – the long process of the incus is missing as it has been eroded. Arrow = Attic cholesteatoma.

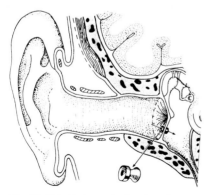

Fig. 10. Ventilating tube in place in tympanic membrane.

fold: (1) Expulsion of the tube by regrowth of epithelium from beneath it, i.e. the epithelium covering the medial side of the drum will eventually cover the inner side of the perforation and 'push' the ventilating tube out. (2) The tube will be expelled by migration of the drum epithelium towards the external canal. The latter is a normal continuous phenomenon, part of the clearance process of the external canal squamous epithelium. Thus, the inserted tube can be left till spontaneously expelled. There are various claims that certain tubes can bring about 'permanent' aeration [67] – which is important in stubborn cases – but they have not been well substantiated.

As most middle ear effusions will clear spontaneously [68, 69] and as there is so far no concrete indication that the effusion is itself harmful, our treatment should be directed to restoration of hearing loss [70]. *There is so far no indication that introduction of the ventilating tubes prevents any of the long-term undesirable states which are seen in obstinate cases of SOM (atelectasis, perforation, cholesteatoma).*

Children, who have a greater loss than 25 dB in *both ears* – and who do not show any indication of spontaneous clearance of the effusion, should therefore be treated. It should be taken into consideration how much their condition disturbs their schooling – at the same time it is usually advisable to wait at least several weeks before resorting to surgical treatment, and see whether a spontaneous cure has not come about. Unilateral hearing loss may be left untreated, unless it becomes bothersome to the patient. It is also good medicine to take into account recurrent episodes of acute otitis media – this increases the indication for middle ear drainage. In such cases, the condition should be viewed as microabscesses – temporarily 'sterilized' by antibiotics – which may flare up periodically until drained. Drainage in these ears will be accomplished best by suctioning the exudate and leaving a ventilating tube in place.

At the same time, one should remember that this treatment like any other, is not devoid of complications. I would therefore suggest introduction of such ventilating grommet in one ear only. This will relieve hearing loss and the effusion in the *other ear* will usually clear with time. Such policy will lessen the occurrence of tympanosclerosis, which are pathological intra-tympanic deposits, seen more often in drums in which a ventilating tube has been inserted, than in others.

Usually, once a ventilating tube has been introduced, the effusion clears through the Eustachian tube within hours; this occurs whether the effusion is aspirated or not [42]. This suggests, among others, that the Eustachian tube is not organically blocked and that the mucociliary system is essentially intact. For this reason, introduction of urea [71] into the middle ear, which breaks the secondary intermolecular bonds and facilitates aspiration of the mucus is really unnecessary. Exceptionally, satisfactory clearance does not occur and an exudate (bacteriologically sterile or not) continues to pulsate from the ventilating tube. This indicates active inflammation which, however, does disappear at times (with or without antibiotics) after an interval of several days, but not always. In the latter cases, the attic and antrum are filled with granulation tissue which, unless removed, will continue to produce an exudate, which might become reinfected. The space occupied by these granulation tissues is not large as mastoids in SOM patients are usually underdeveloped and hypocellular. It is these cases which require a simple atticomastoidectomy – cleaning up all the granulation tissue, but conserving *all* middle ear structures and the middle ear frame (i.e. attic and posterior walls). The patients who require such an operation are few, but in their case, this is the treatment of choice.

There are claims that in the treatment of SOM 'anti-allergic' treatment is rewarding, including administration of antihistamines, corticoids, 'anticongestants' and desensitisation to one or another 'antigen'. However, there is no evidence that SOM is an allergic disease in the sense of it being a response to some foreign allergen or antigen. Any 'treatment' may appear to be beneficial since spontaneous clearance of the effusion eventually occurs in the vast majority of the children. Frequent and routine politzerization (forced middle ear ventilation through the nose with a special balloon) probably belongs also in this category. Lastly, antibiotic treatment is of course of no use whatsoever and contraindicated.

Follow-up of SOM is of importance, and especially of the obstinate cases – as in a small but significant number – the Eustachian tube function does not return to normal, and complications may develop, i.e. atelectasis, central perforation, and even cholesteatomas, and these will require special treatment.

Conclusions

Altogether, the evolution of thought concerning SOM has gone a long way since the day of the mechanistic concept of 'closure' of the Eustachian tube, causing an intratympanic *ex vacuo* negative pressure 'which results in a transudate and retracted drum'. Information obtained over the last two decades shows SOM to be an inflammatory process, the middle ear lining presenting an inflammatory reaction like other respiratory mucosas. The added specific condition in the middle ear is that this inflammatory process happens at times in an under-aerated 'pocket' (the middle ear) – wich bestows its special character: i.e. mucus cell metaplasia and clearance deficiency of mucus. This process is mostly transitory and benign, calling at times for no action. Yet, when hearing is significantly impaired, the ears should be ventilated surgically. A *small* proportion of these patients in whom ventilation will continue to be deficient should be viewed with concern, followed up and treated appropriately, as they may later develop atelectasis, central perforations, and possibly cholesteatoma. While many aspects of SOM have become clarified in the last two decades, its hard core, i.e. the understanding and measurement of the Eustachian tube function and resulting middle ear aeration, is yet to come [72].

References

1   GOODHILL, V. and HOLCOMB, E. E.: The relation of auditory response to the viscosity of tympanic fluids. Acta oto-lar. *49:* 38–46 (1958).

2   SUEHS, O. W.: Chronic secretory otitis media. J. Med. Ass. Geo. *45:* 499–506 (1956).

3   HANTMAN, I.: Secretory otitis media. Archs Otolar. *38:* 561–573 (1943).

4   COHEN, D. and SADÉ, J.: Hearing in secretory otitis media. Can. J. Otolar. *1:* 27–29 (1972).

5   KAPUR, Y. P.: Serous otitis media in children. Archs Otolar. *79:* 38–48 (1964).

6   COHEN, D.: The natural history of serous otitis media; MD thesis, Jerusalem (1968).

7   KOKKO, E.: Chronic secretory otitis media in children. Acta oto-lar. Suppl. *327* (1974).

8   LIN, S. Y.; LANG, R.; LIM, D. J., and BIRCK, H. G.: Microorganisms in chronic otitis media with effusion. Ann. Otol. Rhinol. Lar. *85:* suppl. 25, pp. 245–300 (1976).

9   SENTURIA, B. H.; GESSERT, C. F.; CARR, C. D., and BAUMANN, E. S.: Studies concerned with tubotympanitis. Ann. Otol. Rhinol. Lar. *67:* 440–467 (1958).

10 TILLES, J. G., KLEIN, J. O., JAO, R. L., HASLAM, J. E.; FEINGOLD, M.; GELLIS, S. S., and FINLAND, M.: Acute otitis media in children. New Engl. J. Med. *277:* 613–618 (1967).

11 GWALTNEY, J. M.: Virology of middle ear. Ann. Otol. Rhinol. Lar. *80:* 365–371) (1971).

12 HARVEY, R. M.: Environmental factors in glue ear. J. Lar. Otol. *89:* 73–77 (1975).

13 LIM, D. J.; LIN, S. Y.; SCHRAM, J., and BIRCK, H. G.: Immunoglobulin E in chronic middle ear effusion. Ann. Otol. Rhinol. Lar. *85:* suppl. 25, pp. 117–124 (1976).

14 WRIGHT, I. and KAPADIA, R.: The cytology of 'glue ear'. J. Otol. Rhinol. Lar. *83:* 367–376 (1969).

15 VERED, J.; ELIEZER, N., and SADÉ, J.: Biochemical characterisation of middle ear effusions. Ann. Otol. Rhinol. Lar. *81:* 394–401 (1972).

16 SADÉ, J.: The muco-ciliary system in relation to middle ear pathology and senso-

neural loss. CIBA Found. Symp. Sensoneural Hearing Loss, pp. 79–99 (Churchill, London 1970).

17   MOGI, G. and MONJO, S.: Middle ear effusion – analysis of protein contents. Ann. Otol. Rhinol. Lar. *81:* 99–106 (1972).

18   MEYER, F. A.: Comparison of structural glycoproteins from mucus of different sources. Eur. J. Biochem. (submitted).

19   SENTURIA, B. H.; GESSERT, C. F.; CARR, C. D., and BAUMANN, E. S.: Middle ear effusions: causes and treatment. Am. Acad. Ophthal. Otol. *64:* 60–72 (1960).

20   SADÉ, J.: Middle ear mucosa. Archs Otolar. *84:* 137–143 (1966).

21   SADÉ, J.: Ciliary activity and middle ear clearance. Archs Otolar. *86:* 128–135 (1967).

22   SADÉ, J.; ELIEZER, N.; SILBERBERG, A., and NEVO, A.: The role of mucus in transport by cilia. Am. Rev. resp. Dis. *102:* 48–52 (1970).

23   SADÉ, J.; MEYER, F. A.; KING, M., and SILBERBERG, A.: Clearance of middle ear effusions by the mucociliary system. Acta oto-lar. *79:* 277–282 (1975).

24   CARLSON, L. A. and LOKK, T.: Protein studies of transudatees of the middle ear. Scand. J. clin. Lab. Invest. *7:* 43–48 (1955).

25   GESSERT, C. F.; BAUMANN, E. S., and SENTURIA, B. H.: Middle ear effusions produced experimentally in dogs. Ann. Otol. Rhinol. Lar. *68:* 1028–1037 (1959).

26   VELTRI, R. W. and SPRINKLE, P. M.: Serous otitis media. Ann. Otol. Rhinol. Lar. *82:* 297–302 (1973).

27   MOGI, G.; HONJO, S.; MAEDA, S., and YOSHIDA, T.: Secretory immunoglobulin A in middle ear effusions. Ann. Otol. Rhinol. Lar. *82:* 302–311 (1973).

28   PAPARELLA, M. M. and DITO, W. R.: Enzyme studies in serous otitis media. Archs Otolar. *79:* 393–398 (1964).

29   JUHN, S. K.; HUFF, J. S., and PAPARELLA, M. M.: Lactate dehydrogenase activity and isoenzyme patterns in serous middle ear effusions. Ann. Otol. Rhinol. Lar. *82:* 192 to 196 (1973).

30   JUHN, S. K.; HUFF, J. S., and PAPARELLA, M. M.: Biochemical analysis of middle ear effusions. Ann. Otol. Rhinol. Lar. *80:* 347–354 (1971).

31   PALVA, T.; RAUNIO, V., and MONSIANEN, R.: Secretory otitis media: protein and enzyme analysis. Ann. Otol. Rhinol. Lar. *83:* suppl. 11, pp. 35–43 (1974).

32   LIM, D. J.: Functional morphology of the mucosa of the middle ear and eustachian tube. Ann. Otol. Rhinol. Lar. *85:* suppl. 25, pp. 36–44 (1976).

33   HUSSL, B. and LIM., D. J.: Experimental middle ear effusions: an immunofluorescent study. Ann. Otol. Rhinol. Lar. *83:* 332–343 (1974).

34   PALVA, T.; HOLOPAINEN, E., and KARMA, P.: Protein and cellular pattern of glue ear and secretions. Ann. Otol. Rhinol. Lar. *85:* suppl. 25, pp. 103–119 (1976).

35   LIM, D.; LIN, Y. S., and BIRCK, H.: Secretory lyzozyme of the human middle ear mucosa. Ann. Otol. Rhinol. Lar. *85:* 50–61 (1976).

36   BERNSTEIN, J.; TOMASI, T. B., and OGRA, P.: The immunochemistry of middle ear effusions. Archs Otolar. *99:* 320–326 (1974).

37   MOGI, G.; HONJO, S.; MEADA, S.; YOSHIDA, T., and WATANABE, N.: Immunoglobulin E in middle ear effusions. Ann. Otol. Rhinol. Lar. *83:* 393–397 (1974).

38   DIAMANT, M.: Abuse and timing of use of antibiotics in acute otitis media. Archs Otolar. *100:* 226–232 (1974).

39   SADÉ, J. and BERCO, E.: Atelectasis and secretory otitis media. Ann. Otol. Rhinol. Lar. *85:* suppl. 25, pp. 66–73 (1976).

40 BROOKS, D.N.: School screening for middle ear effusions. Ann. Otol. Rhinol. Lar. *85:* suppl. 25, pp. 223–228 (1976).

41 SADÉ, J.; HALEVY, A., and HADAS, E.: Clearance of middle ear effusions and middle ear pressures. Ann. Otol. Rhinol. Lar. *85:* suppl. 25, pp. 58–62 (1976).

42 BUCKINGHAM, R.A. and FERRER, J.L.: Middle ear pressures in eustachian tube malfunction. Laryngoscope *83:* 1585–1593 (1973).

43 DAWES, J.D.K.: The aetiology and sequelae of exudative otitis media. J. Lar. Otol. *84:* 583–610 (1970).

44 BIRCK, H.G. and MRAVEC, J.J.: Myringostomy for middle ear effusions. Ann. Otol. Rhinol. Lar. *85:* suppl. 25, pp. 263–267 (1976).

45 SADÉ, J.: Pathology and pathogenesis of serous otitis media. Archs Otolar. *84:* 297–305 (1966).

46 MAWSON, S.R. and FAGAN, P.: Tympanic effusions in children. J. Lar. Otol. *86:* 105–119 (1972).

47 HOLMQUIST, J. and RENNWALL, U.: Eustachian tube function in secretory otitis media. Archs Otolar. *99:* 59–61 (1974).

48 PARADISE, J. and BLUESTONE, C.D.: Diagnosis and management of ear disease in cleft palate infants. Trans. Am. Acad. Ophthal. Otol. *73:* 709–714 (1969).

49 YULES, R.: Hearing in cleft palate children. Archs Otolar. *91:* 319–323 (1970).

50 HOLBORROW, C.: Conductive deafness associated with the cleft-palate deformity. Proc. R. Soc. Med. *55:* 305–307 (1962).

51 STEVENS, D.: Serous otitis as a cause of catarrhal deafness in childhood. Lancet *1958:* July 5th, pp. 22–24.

52 INGELSTED, S.; JOHNSON, B., and RUNDCRANZ, H.: Gas tension and pH in middle ear effusions. Ann. Otol. Rhinol. Lar. *84:* 198–203 (1975).

53 SADÉ, J.; DRUCKER, I.; WEISMAN, Z., and NEVO, A.: Effects of environmental factors on respiratory epithelial. Air pollution and the lung, pp. 141–148 (Wiley & Sons, Toronto 1975).

54 SADÉ, J. and WEISMAN, Z.: Middle ear mucosa and secretory media. To be published in Proc. 5th Shambough Workshop on Microsurgery (Aesculapius, 1977).

55 DRUCKER, I.; WEISMAN, Z., and SADÉ, J.: Tissue culture of human adult adenoids and of middle ear mucosa. Ann. Otol. Rhinol. Lar. *85:* 327–334 (1976).

56 SADÉ, J. and WEISMAN, Z.: The phenotypic expression of middle ear mucosa. To be published in Cholesteatoma – Proc. 1st Int. Conf. Cholesteatoma (Aesculapius, 1977).

57 LIM, D.J. and BIRCK, H.: Ultrastructural pathology of the middle ear mucosa in serous otitis media. Ann. Otol. Rhinol. Lar. *80:* 838–854 (1971).

58 HENTZER, E.: Ultrastructure of the middle ear mucosa in secretory otitis media. Acta Oto-lar. *73:* 394–401 (1972).

59 DEMOURA, L.F.P. and HAYDEN, R.C.: Pathology of secretory otitis media. Henry Ford Hosp. med. J. *17:* 25–34 (1969).

60 BAK-PEDERSEN, K. and TOS, M.: The mucous glands in chronic secretory otitis media. Acta Oto-lar. *72:* 14–27 (1971).

61 GUNDERSEN, T. and GLUCK, E.: The middle ear mucosa in serous otitis media. Archs Otolar. *96:* 40–44 (1972).

62 SADÉ, J. and HALEVY, A.: The natural history of chronic otitis media. J. Lar. Otol. *90:* 743–751 (1976).

63 Fabricius, H.F.: Hearing investigations of school children in North Trondelay County. J.Oslo City Hosp. *18:* 3–44 (1968).

64 Mackinnon, D.M.: The sequel to myringotomy for exudative otitis media. J.Lar. Otol. *85:* 773–793 (1971).

65 Sheehy, J.L.: Collar button tube for chronic serous otitis. Am.Acad.Ophthal.Otol. *68:* 888–889 (1964).

66 Fenerstein, S.S.: Surgery of serous otitis media. Laryngoscope *76:* 686–708 (1966).

67 Silverstein, H.: Permanent middle ear aeration. Archs Otolar. *91:* 313–318 (1970).

68 Cowan, D.L. and Brown, M.J.K.M.: Seromucinous otitis media and its sequelae. J.Laryng.Otol. *88:* 1237–1247 (1974).

69 Gottschalk, H.G.: Further experience with controlled middle ear inflation in the treatment of serous otitis. Eye Ear Throat mthl. *45:* 49–51 (1966).

70 Proud, G.O.: Middle ear effusions. Trans.Pac.Coast Oto-Ophth.Soc. *68:* 189–192 (1967).

71 Bauer, F.: Treatment of 'glue ear' by intratympanic injection of urea. J.Lar.Otol. *82:* 717–722 (1968).

72 Sadé, J.: The biopathology of secretory otitis media. Ann.Otol.Rhinol.Lar. *83:* suppl.11, pp.59–71 (1974).

J.Sadé, MD, The Meir Hospital Kfar-Saba, The Weizmann Institute, *Rehovot* (Israel)

Adv. Oto-Rhino-Laryng., vol. 23, pp. 22–28 (Karger, Basel 1978)

Hazards of Ventilation Tubes

Moshe Harell and John J. Shea

Shea Clinic, Memphis, Tenn.

Serous otitis media has its peak incidence in early childhood, in the age group of 3–7 years. There are several factors which contribute to the creation of this problem, and their relative etiologic importance is difficult to assess.

Many children have recurrent upper respiratory infections, and/or nasal allergy, which increases secretion and produces mucosal edema. The condition is especially severe in this age group as, until the age of 7, the Eustachian tube lumen is small and the nasopharyngeal orifice is surrounded by lymphoid tissue. In some instances, the lumen may be obstructed by lymphoid follicles in the tubal mucosa *per se*. In children, the tube lies quite low, in the plane of the base of the skull, and its cartilages and intrinsic muscles are still undeveloped [9, 19, 20]. Blocking of the Eustachian tube causes negative pressure build-up in the middle ear cleft: this is, in turn, a direct, as well as an indirect, cause of serous otitis media. Transudation and bleeding are directly related to the negative pressure, whereas mucosal changes (glandular hypertrophy, edema) have an indirect relation to it. The condition, if untreated, can cause serious later complications, such as adhesive otitis, ossicular destruction, cholesteatoma, and chronic suppurative ear disease.

Treatment should be aimed at removing the fluid and at restoring normal ventilation and pressure in the middle ear. This, along with the treatment of etiologic factors, such as infections or allergies, will bring about the return to normal function of the middle ear and eustachian mucosa, provided that the mucosal changes are still reversible, and the treatment is continued long enough. In other words, early diagnosis and treatment of serous otitis media, before permanent damage has occurred, is essential.

Ventilation of the middle ear by somewhat crude methods (such as partial excision of the tympanic membrane, introduction of 'cannulas', 'eyelets', and various foreign bodies through the tympanic membrane) was attempted as early as the beginning of the 19th century. Those procedures were abandoned for almost 100 years, due to the infections, dislodgings, and closures resulting in failures. It was not until 1954, when the modern ventilation tube was introduced by ARMSTRONG [1], that the idea of artificial aeration of the middle ear gained almost ubiquitous acceptance. Since then, the dimensions of its use in this country have made this surgical procedure one of the most frequently performed operations. A prominent otologist says that he has inserted as many as 15,000 tubes, and many others are not far behind. The extravagant popularity of the tube has led to its widespread use by general practitioners and pediatricians in a variety of situations, including its insertion in infants' ears. With a few exceptions, use of ventilation tubes by others than otolaryngologists is, as a general rule, to be deplored.

There is a general consensus that the ventilation tube has its place in the modern treatment of serous otitis media. However, to quote ARMSTRONG [1] himself: 'This method is not presented as a panacea in the management of secretory otitis media. It has been used only in chronic cases that have resisted treatment.' And again, 14 years later, in 1968, ARMSTRONG [2] warns, 'Tubes have limitations: they extrude, they become plugged, and they may incite complications.'

The overuse of ventilation tubes leads to the inevitable conclusion that many physicians seem to be unaware of the limitations and hazards of the tubes. There also seems to be a widespread unawareness of the existence of other ways to successfully treat the majority of serous otitis media cases in childhood. Many authorities share the view that myringotomy and autoinflation, along with medical treatment, is at least as effective as ventilation tubes, if not superior to them, in the majority of cases. DONALDSON's statement (as quoted by ARMSTRONG [2]), may seem surprising, but is concise and very true: 'The tube is an admission of failure after allergy, sinus infection, adenoids, etc., have been maximally treated.' We would add to this list myringotomy and autoinflation.

The overuse of tubes can be explained also by the immediate, positive effect demonstrated by hearing gain. However, in long-term follow-up studies, there is no difference in recurrence rate and hearing levels between tube-treated children and those treated with myringotomy [12]. The difference, regrettably, is in a higher rate of complications in the tube patients. Thus, the short-term effect of improved hearing while the tubes are *in situ*

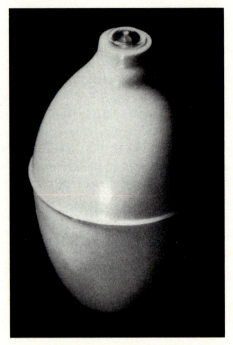

Fig. 1. Mathes Inflation Bulb. The Mathes bulbs, identification 13 mini-politzer-bulb, are sold by The De Vilbiss Company, Medical Products Division, Somerset, Pa.

tends to divert attention from two important problems: (a) Most tubes are extruded before the pathologic changes in the middle ear and Eustachian mucosa have reversed. This causes a high recurrence rate. It has been noted that cases most likely to benefit from tubes are those which are most likely to quickly extrude them, because of excessive epithelial proliferation [12, 15]. (b) Long-term tube therapy, whether by reinsertion or by non-extruded tubes, frequently causes serious complications. As a result, the otologist is faced with the dilemma that long-term tube therapy is essential for cure, while on the other hand, prolonged treatment leads to complications.

The most common long-term complications are those involving changes in the appearance and structure of the tympanic membrane. These can be divided into two major groups: (1) tympanosclerotic changes, and (2) scarring and atrophic changes.

Tympanosclerotic Changes

The incidence of tympanosclerotic changes increases with the length of follow-up. During a course of 5–6 years follow-up, it has been reported in as much as 30–33 % of tube-treated ears [15, 16]. Kokko [13] and Tos and Poulsen [22] reported lower figures: 14–15 % on long-term follow-ups. Histologically, tympanosclerotic change appears as hyaline degeneration of connective tissue in the drum, forming calcium-containing plaques. The incidence of tympanosclerosis in ears treated without tubes is reported to be 3–8 % [13, 15]. Cowan and Brown [5] have shown that hearing loss is greater in ears with tympanosclerosis than in those without. Thus, there is evidence that the use of tubes predisposes to tympanosclerosis, which is a cause for further hearing loss.

Scarring and Atrophic Changes

Reports of this complication in tube treated ears vary between 35 and 79 % [3, 8, 22]. Atrophy is associated with loss of the middle layer of the drum, as was demonstrated by Kerr and Smyth [11]; in addition, the tympanic membrane around the tube was thickened. This very high incidence of degenerative changes in tube treated ears is, at least partially, directly related to the tube *per se*, although some blame the disease for it. Kilby *et al.* [12] treated bilateral serous otitis media by tube insertion in one ear and simple myringotomy in the other. In a 2-year follow-up, they found 37 % (15 of 41) of scarred and/or atrophic drums in the tubed ears, whereas the myringotomy ears had 12 % (5 of 41).

Surprisingly enough, permanent perforation and cholesteatoma have a relatively low incidence in these cases. In the literature since 1970, cholesteatoma figures range between 1.1 and 5.6 %, and perforations were noted in 1.6–4.5 % in long-term follow-up series. Schuknecht [19] reports three cases of middle ear keratoma, and Pahor [17] recently reported another case of keratoma following tube insertion.

Chronic suppurative otitis media is another complication, the incidence of which is quite variable (0–7.7 % in large series). It seems worthwhile to note that in Armstrong's [2] survey among 320 otolaryngologists on the use of tubes, 70.8 % of the treating physicians attributed the development of suppurative otitis media to tube insertion.

Our experience at the Shea Clinic, a referral center, is somewhat different. During the past 4 years, 17 children (26 ears) were referred to us for treatment of complications resulting from tube insertion. The age range was 2–16 years. Five of them had tube insertion more than once (1 child had had 10 consecutive yearly tube placements, starting at the age of 6).

In 12 ears (46 %) the problem was suppurative otitis media, 6 of which grew Pseudomonas on cultures. Two ears (8 %) showed extensive granulations on the drums, around the tubes. Five ears (19 %) had to undergo mastoidectomy, and in 2 (8 %) cholesteatoma was found. Five ears (19 %) had persistent dry perforation, 4 of which had myringoplasty for its closure. Atrophic, scarred drums were found in 3 ears (12 %). As already stated, these data represent a selected group, because they are referred, pre-treated cases.

An extreme example of ventilation tube complication is an 8-year-old boy who had tracheotomy because of severe hypoxia caused by laryngitis and pneumonia [20]. The latter were complications of staphylococcal otitis media following tube insertion for serous otitis media. He had a previous successful repair of his cleft palate. As a result of the severe hypoxia, the child suffered brain damage. His hearing improved after myringotomy, and stayed stable due to autoinflation that he was taught to practice daily.

Most authors agree that the average duration of the tube in the tympanic membrane is 3–6 months [10, 12, 15, 16, 19]. Obviously, this relatively short period is insufficient for cure of the disease. Cure rates (judged by hearing level) range between 36 and 79 % at several years of follow-ups; however, 23–61 % of the tube-treated ears had to be re-intubated one or more times.

Eustachian tube function rarely, if ever, returns to normal following artificial ventilation by means of tubes [15, 22]. Its functional ability remains compromised in most cases, in spite of apparent clinical 'cure'. Practically, this means proneness to recurrence of serous otitis with or without infection – or, in other words, it means non-causal treatment.

Treatment for serous otitis media at the Shea Clinic consists of aspirating the fluid through myringotomy, in cases of thick, rubbery secretions (so-called 'glue ears'), as well as in cases with thin, profuse fluid. In patients, 3 years or older, who have thin, not-too-extensive fluid, the child and parents are taught to inflate the middle ear with the Mathes bulb. This bulb has a 30-ml volume, and is provided with a valve at the tip to limit the speed of air extruded by squeezing it. The valve end is placed in one nostril, the other nostril is closed, and the patient swallows while gently squeezing the bulb. In addition, antibiotics and antihistamines with decongestants are prescribed when needed. The tonsils are removed only if chronically infected, and the adenoids if very large. In small or uncooperative children, or in resistant and recurrent cases, a ventilation tube is inserted. Even with the tube in place, inflation is continued in cooperative patients. The tube is removed as soon as the middle ear can be inflated with ease, and autoinflation is continued daily for a long period (months to years, depending on the individual case), with periodic check-ups, usually once or twice a year.

Summary

Ventilation tubes are not the treatment of choice in serous otitis media. Conservative measures should be tried first, with simple myringotomy for the evacuation of thick, rubbery fluids. Autoinflation, well tolerated by most children above 3 years of age, should be practiced daily for months to years, under periodic check-ups. Tube insertion should be reserved for younger children, as well as for recurrent and non-responsive cases. These are the cases in which a calculated risk is worth taking, as otherwise the patient is on an ineffective treatment. In those hard-to-manage ears, tubes seem to be justified, as their potential hazards are apparently outnumbered by the complication of untreated or maltreated serous otitis media.

References

1   ARMSTRONG, B.W.: A new treatment for chronic secretory otitis media. Archs Otolar. *59:* 653–654 (1954).
2   ARMSTRONG, B.W.: What your colleagues think of tympanostomy tubes. Laryngoscope *78:* 1303–1313 (1968).
3   BONDING, P. and LORENZEN, E.: Cicatricial changes of the eardrum after treatment with grommets. Acta oto-lar. *75:* 275–276 (1973).
4   BONDING, P. and LORENZEN, E.: Chronic secretory otitis media – long-term results after treatment with grommets. ORL *36:* 227–235 (1974).
5   COWAN, D.L. and BROWN, J.K.M.: Seromucinous otitis media and its sequelae. J.Lar.Otol. *88:* 1237–1247 (1974).
6   FEUERSTEIN, S.S.: Surgery of serous otitis media. Laryngoscope *76:* 686–708 (1966).
7   GOTTSCHALK, G.H.: Serous Otitis. A conservative approach to treatment. Archs Otolar. *96:* 110–112 (1972).
8   GUNDERSEN, T. and TONNING, F.M.: Ventilating tubes in the middle ear. Long-term observations. Archs Otolar. *102:* 198–199 (1976).
9   HOLBOROW, C.: Eustachian tubal function. Archs Otolar. *92:* 624–626 (1970).
10 JONS, C.D. and DONALDSON, J.A.: The artificial eustachian tube. Otolar.Clin.N. Am. *3:* 55–59 (1970).

11   KERR, A.G. and SMYTH, G.D.L.: Secretory otitis media – a temporal bone report. J.Lar.Otol. *87:* 611–614 (1973).
12   KILBY, D.; RICHARDS, S.H., and HART, G.: Grommets and glue ears: two-year results. J.Lar.Otol. *86:* 881–888 (1972).
13   KOKKO, E.: Chronic secretory otitis media in children. A clinical study. Acta oto-lar. Suppl. *327:* 7–44 (1974).
14   LINTHICUM, F.H.: Otitis media: the search for definitive treatment continues. ORL Dig. *38:* 8–9 (1976).
15   MACKINNON, D.M.: The sequel to myringotomy for exudative otitis media. J.Lar. Otol. *85:* 773–793 (1971).
16   MAWSON, S.R. and FAGAN, P.: Tympanic effusions in children. J.Lar.Otol. *86:* 105–119 (1972).
17   PAHOR, A.L.: Intratympanic keratoma following grommet insertion. J.Lar.Otol. *90:* 1155–1157 (1976).
18   RAWLINS, A.G.: The value of self-inflation of the middle ear. Archs Otolar. *69:* 547–548 (1959).
19   SCHUKNECHT, H.F.: Pathology of the ear, pp.254–256 (Harvard University Press, Cambridge 1974).
20   SHEA, J.J.: Autoinflation treatment of serous otitis media in children. J.Tenn.med. Ass. *65:* 104–108 (1972).
21   THOMSON, I.S.D.: Exudative otitis media, grommets and cholesteatoma. J.Lar. Otol. *88:* 947–953 (1974).
22   TOS, M. and POULSEN, G.: Secretory otitis media. Late results of treatment with grommets. Archs Otolar. *102:* 672–675 (1976).
23   TURNER, J.L.: Myringostomy by use of a fixed prosthesis. Laryngoscope *77:* 524–533 (1967).

M.HARELL, MD, Shea Clinic, 1080 Madison Avenue, *Memphis, TN 38104* (USA)

Adv. Oto-Rhino-Laryng., vol. 23, pp. 29–44 (Karger, Basel 1978)

Histopathology of the Middle Ear in Chronic Otitis Media[1]

FRED H. LINTHICUM, jr.

Otologic Medical Group, Inc., and the Ear Research Institute, Los Angeles, Calif.

The introduction of antimicrobials in the early 1940s changed the concept of the etiology of chronic otitis media. It now appears that in most cases the condition begins in childhood or infancy and, unless adequate prophylactic measures are taken, leads to the complications that are so familiar. The underlying problem is one of faulty Eustachian tubal function in infancy and childhood. The failure of the *Eustachian* tube to ventilate the middle ear results in a delayed absorption of mesenchyme in the epitympanum, which can lead to the primary acquired cholesteatoma. Likewise, the failure of ventilation of the middle ear results in a persistent negative pressure, causing a transudate to fill the middle ear and mastoid spaces. This in turn makes the ear very susceptible to recurrent infection by organisms normally tolerated in the nasopharynx but not in the middle ear.

Eustachian tubal malfunction is not necessarily an antecedent of chronic otitis media. Some organisms (Pneumococcus, Streptococcus, and *Hemophilus influenzae*) are capable of directly invading the middle ear without preexisting middle ear effusion and producing necrotizing otitis media (fig. 1). This results in a perforation of the tympanic membrane and possibly destruction of parts of the ossicular chain, particularly the long process of the incus. Fortunately, such complications are rare in the modern era due to the multitude of antimicrobial agents now available. However, occasional cases are still seen where treatment has been delayed and damage occurs.

By far the most common cause of chronic middle ear disease is a persistent middle ear effusion due to faulty Eustachian tubal function. This can lead to a multitude of pathological conditions, including perforation of

[1] The histopathologic material was prepared in the Eccles Temporal Bone Laboratory and reviewed in the Larrabee Microscopy Center of the Ear Research Institute.

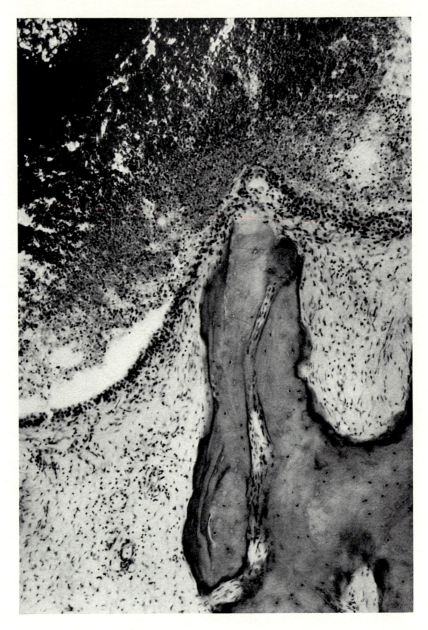

Fig. 1. Acute necrotizing otitis media. Pus fills the air spaces and there is beginning hyperplasia of the mucosa. × 110.

the tympanic membrane, ossicular chain destruction, primary or secondary acquired cholesteatoma, or cholesterol granuloma.

Tympanic Membrane and Ossicular Destruction

The persistent middle ear effusion that becomes repeatedly infected, usually with Staphylococcus, may eventually lead to a perforation of the tympanic membrane and destruction of the lenticular process of the incus. The presence of a perforation in the tympanic membrane makes the patient more susceptible to recurrent middle ear infections. Water may easily enter the middle ear, carrying with it debris from the external auditory canal. This debris can act as a foreign body and lead to recurrent suppuration. Due to the perforation in the tympanic membrane, the middle ear cleft is no longer a closed system, so that any increase in pressure in the nasopharynx may force mucus-bearing saphrophytic organisms from the nasopharynx into the middle ear cleft where they are no longer saprophytes but pathogens. Repeated episodes will result in destruction of parts of the ossicular chain, particularly the long process of the incus and more rarely the stapedial crura.

Middle Ear Effusion

Failure of the Eustachian tube to open during the act of swallowing will result in absorption of the gases in the middle ear. Swallowing occurs approximately every 3 min in adults and more frequently in children. The result is a transudate to replace the negative pressure. During the early stages of the condition, the mucosa undergoes little change (fig. 2). If the condition is chronic, eventually there is hyperplasia and metaplasia of the middle ear mucosa (fig. 3). In the normal middle ear, the only secretory epithelium is in the anterior half of the middle ear cleft, including a small portion of the mucosa on the medial side of the tympanic membrane. In chronic middle ear effusions, the mucosa undergoes a metaplasia to a secretory ciliated epithelium. There is submucosal connective tissue hypertrophy. SADE [1] has demonstrated mucus-secreting glands in such ears. The disease has now become the true secretory otitis media (fig. 4). Ventilation of the middle ear with a transtympanic tube will usually result in a reversal of the pathologic process and the mucosa will assume its normal microscopic appearance.

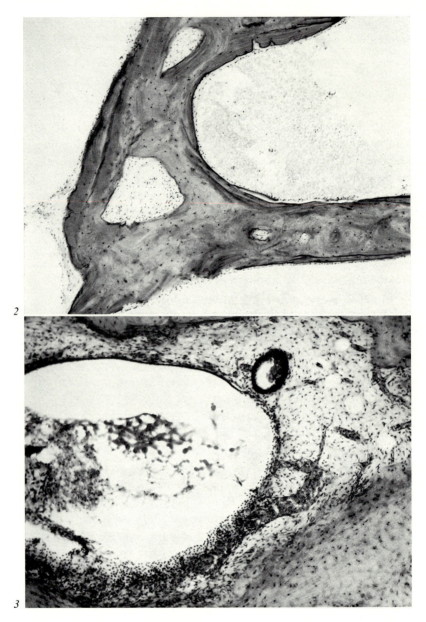

Fig. 2. Early stage of middle ear effusion. A few pus cells are seen in the fluid, but rarely can a positive culture be obtained. × 92.

Fig. 3. Intermediate stage of middle ear effusion. There is hyperplasia of the submucosa and increased vascularity. × 100.

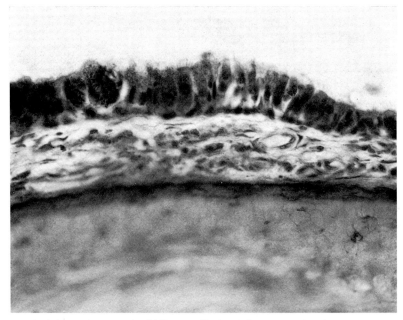

Fig.4. Advanced stage of middle ear effusion. The mucosa has become secretory ciliated columnar. This microphoto is from the head of the malleus, which is ordinarily covered by low cuboidal epithelium. × 410.

Tympanosclerosis

Tympanosclerosis is apparently the end result of a vasculitis produced by chronic or recurrent otitis media. Chronic middle ear effusion with or without infection will result in a submucosal hypertrophy of fibrous tissue[2], If the blood supply is inadequate, hyalinization, calcification, and eventually ossification may occur. Tympanosclerosis has been described as a destructive process [3]. However, evaluation of temporal bones in the Ear Research Institute Eccles and Larrabee Laboratories indicates that it is not. Tympanosclerosis may occur in the tympanic membrane, or anywhere in the middle ear, due to decreased vascularity (fig.5, 6). Were it a destructive process, one would expect it to destroy the crura of the stapes, the most delicate osseous structures in the middle ear. However, the stapedial crura and capitulum may be enveloped by tympanosclerosis without evidence of

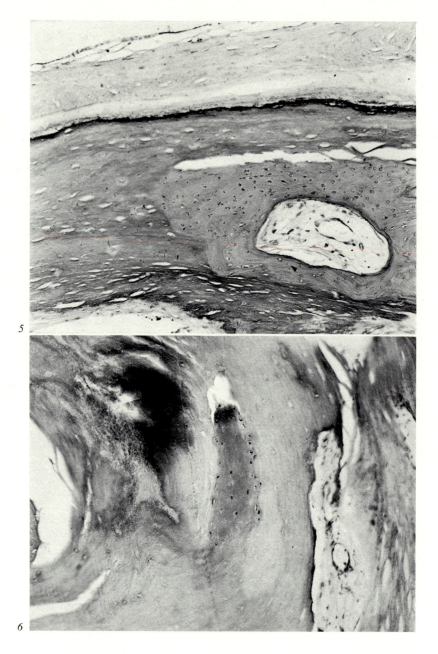

Fig.5. Tympanosclerosis in the tympanic membrane. Note actual bone formation and the presence of a marrow space in the bone. × 110.

Fig.6. Tympanosclerosis from the promontory. Hyalinization, calcification, and ossification are evident. × 110.

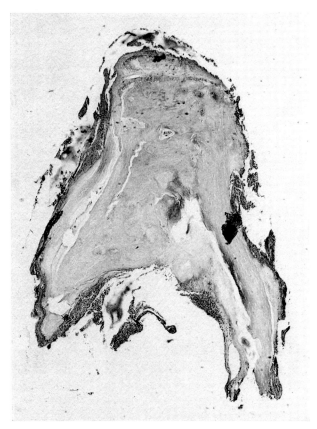

Fig. 7. Capitulum and crura of the stapes enveloped by the tympanosclerosis. × 51.

destruction (fig. 7). Apparently what was previously thought to be destruction by the tympanosclerotic process was actually preexisting bone destruction. These areas became replaced by fibrous tissue and due to the impaired vascularity underwent hyalinization, calcification, and eventually ossification. Experience has taught us, however, that removal of tympanosclerotic plaques about the ossicles will not necessarily result in a persistent hearing improvement. The blood supply has already been impaired, and even if the tympanosclerosis is removed, it is replaced by fibrous tissue which is still lacking an adequate blood supply and hence the process begins again, regardless of whether there is recurrent infection.

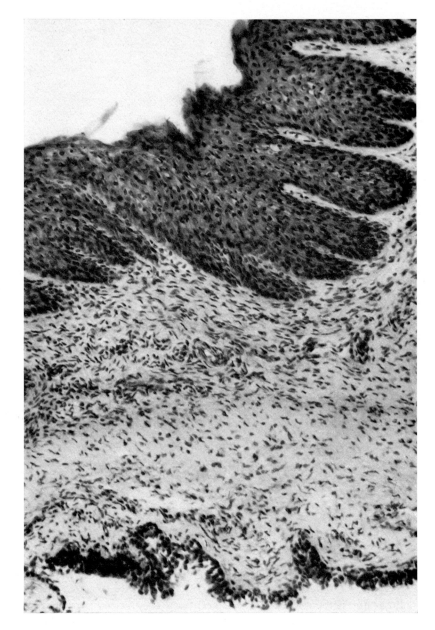

Fig.8. Rete pegs extending into the mesenchyme of the pars flaccida. At the top is the squamous epithelium and rete pegs. At the bottom of the picture is the middle ear mucosa. × 106.

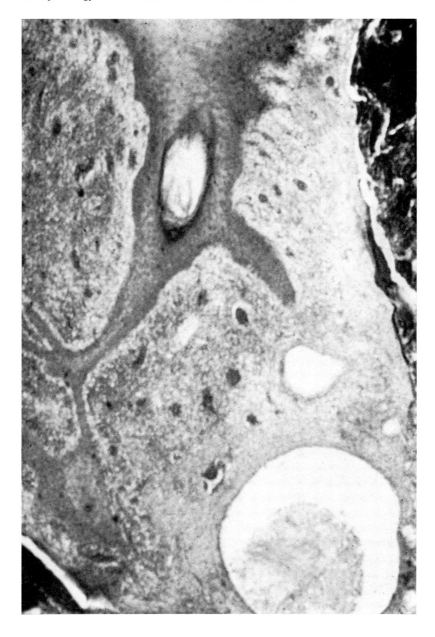

Fig.9. Squamous epithelium extending into the unresolved mesenchyme and the beginning of the formation of a cyst. × 33.

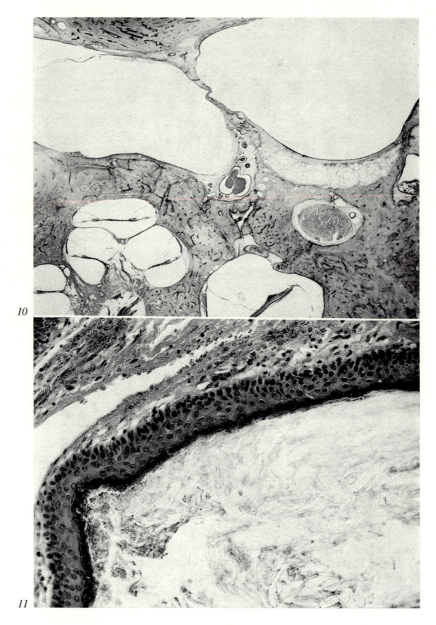

Fig. 10. Atrophic retracted tympanic membrane. × 7.0.

Fig. 11. Matrix of the cholesteatoma demonstrating desquamation and accumulation of debris. × 400.

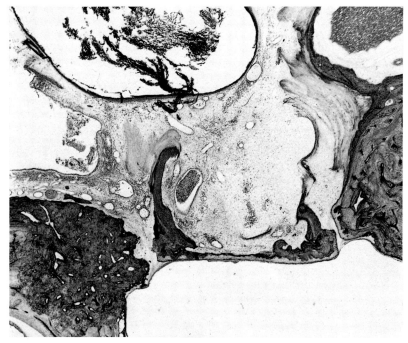

Fig. 12. Secondary acquired cholesteatoma that has eroded the incus and capitulum of the stapes. Also evident in this picture is some tympanosclerosis adjacent to the facial nerve and an otosclerotic focus in the anterior portion of the oval window. × 32.

Primary Acquired Cholesteatoma

The pars flaccida of the tympanic membrane contains no fibrous layer beneath the squamous epithelium. Early in life, should the mesenchyme in the epitympanum fail to absorb because of faulty Eustachian tubal function, the rete pegs of the squamous epithelium can invade it (fig. 8). These rete pegs can become isolated and begin the formation of a cyst as squamous epithelium desquamates (fig. 9) [4]. There is not necessarily any antecedent infection. The cyst continues to enlarge, destroying the ossicles and bone of the epitympanum and aditus and may not become apparent until the child is found to have a conductive hearing loss. In its early stages, the primary acquired cholesteatoma does not block the aditus or antrum and therefore pneumatization of the mastoid develops normally. Later, as the cholesteatoma expands, it will invade the now pneumatized mastoid and produce the so-called cholesteatosis, which has invaded the entire well-pneumatized mastoid air cell system.

Secondary Acquired Cholesteatoma

Repeated episodes of otitis media or insertion of ventilation tubes can cause destruction of the fibrous layer of the pars tensa of the tympanic membrane. The negative pressure that originally led to the middle ear effusion will cause the atrophic portion of the tympanic membrane to be retracted into the middle ear, especially in the posterior superior quadrant (fig. 10). As desquamation occurs in this retraction pocket, it begins to accumulate and further enhances the development of a cholesteatoma sac (fig. 11). These habitually migrate into the epitympanum through the posterior superior quadrant of the tympanic membrane and occasionally into the anterior superior quadrant. This type of cholesteatoma is located below the posterior or anterior malleal ligaments (fig. 12). Cholesteatomas, whether they be primary acquired, secondary acquired, or congenital, destroy bone before soft tissues. It has been demonstrated that there are proteolytic enzymes secreted by the matrix that have an affinity for bone rather than soft tissue. It is for this reason that cholesteatomas may cause extensive destruction of the ossicular chain, otic capsule, and mastoid cells before becoming manifest.

Cholesterol Granuloma

A long-standing middle ear effusion can lead to cholesterol granuloma. This occurs if there ist bleeding into the middle ear effusion. The bleeding is probably secondary to the persistent negative middle ear pressure and results in rupture of the small blood vessels in the middle ear mucosa.

Blood is tolerated in the middle ear for short periods of time. Obviously, in all stapedectomy procedures, tympanoplasties, and after skull fractures, there is bleeding into the middle ear, but the blood is evacuated through the Eustachian tube. However, when bleeding occurs into a chronic middle ear effusion and the blood remains there for many weeks or months, erythrocytes degenerate and liberate cholesterol [5]. The cholesterol acts as a foreign body and stimulates the formation of granulation tissue (fig. 13). The middle ear mucosa undergoes a metaplasia to a ciliated secretory type. Eventually, the granulation tissue begins to surround the middle ear effusion and produce cysts (fig. 14). These cysts contain cholesterol crystals that appear surgically as gold flecks. Eventually, the granulation tissue changes to fibrous tissue and leads to the completely fibrotic middle ear and mastoid, for which as yet

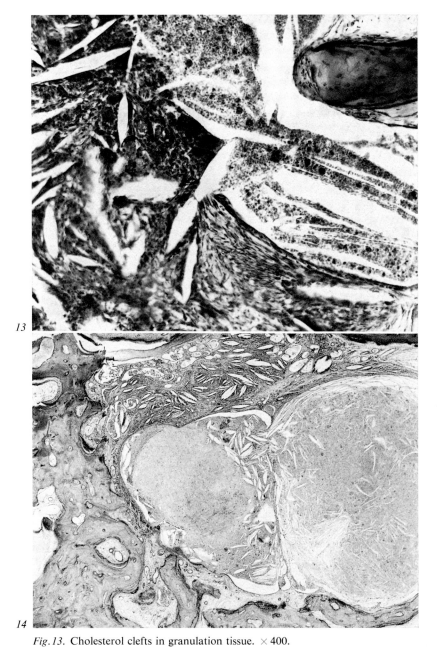

Fig.13. Cholesterol clefts in granulation tissue. × 400.

Fig.14. Middle ear effusion containing cholesterol clefts and surrounded by proliferating granuloma. × 7.5.

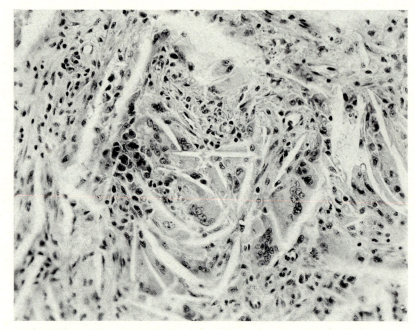

Fig. 15. Cholesterol granuloma removed from a mastoid in which the aditus was blocked by a cholesteatoma. × 400.

no surgical correction has been found. Typically, the tympanic membrane appears opaque and immobile.

Evidence that cholesterol granuloma is not an inflammatory disease is that it can occur in a mastoid cavity in which there has been an obliteration of the antrum by cholesteatoma (fig. 15). The two conditions may coexist but are not related. The cholesteatoma is due to invagination of squamous epithelium into the inner ear or epitympanum; the cholesterol granuloma is due to obliteration of the necessary air supply to the middle ear and mastoid air cell system.

Atelectatic Ear

Should the Eustachian tube begin to function in a patient who has had recurrent otitis media, there will no longer be a persistent negative pressure.

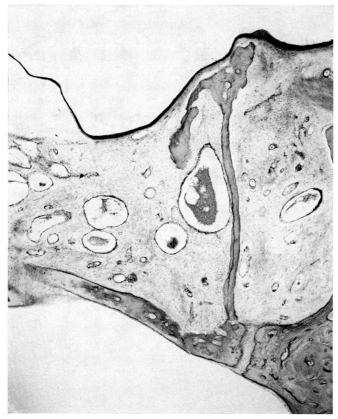

Fig. 16. Spontaneous myringostapediopexy produced by the retraction of atrophic tympanic membrane. The anterior crus of the stapes has been destroyed by the preexisting inflammatory process. × 40.

However, previous destruction of the fibrous layer may have caused portions of the tympanic membrane to become atrophic. The preexisting negative pressure caused this to be retracted into the middle ear and adherent to the promontory, but since there is no longer negative pressure, a secondary acquired cholesteatoma does not form. We therefore see the patients who have the retracted atrophic drum which may become in contact with the stapes after having destroyed the long process of the incus and lead to a myringostapediopexy (fig. 16).

References

1 SADÉ, J.: Pathology and pathogenesis of serous otitis media. Archs Otolar. *84:* 79–87 (1966).
2 SHEEHY, J.L., and HOUSE, W.F.: Tympanosclerosis. Archs Otolar. *76:* 151–157 (1962).
3 HARRIS, I. and WEISS, L.: Tympanosclerosis – Superficial and invasive. 66th Annu. Meet. Am. Academy of Ophthalmology and Otolaryngology, Chicago 1961.
4 RUEDI, L.: Die Pathogenese und die Behandlung der Mittelohrcholesteatome. Mschr. Ohrenheilk. *99:* 153–169 (1965).
5 SHEEHY, J.L.; LINTHICUM, F.H., jr., and GREENFIELD, E.C.: Chronic serous mastoiditis, idiopathic hemotympanum and cholesterol granuloma of the mastoid. Laryngoscope *79:* 1189–1217 (1969).

Dr. F.H. LINTHICUM, jr., The Otologic Medical Group Inc. and the Ear Research Institute, 256 South Lake Street, *Los Angeles, CA 90057* (USA)

Adv. Oto-Rhino-Laryng., vol. 23, pp. 45–57 (Karger, Basel 1978)

Management of Noncholesteatomatous Suppurative Middle Ear Disease in Children

T. PALVA and E. HOLOPAINEN

Department of Otolaryngology, University of Helsinki, Helsinki

Introduction

The disease entity – noncholesteatomatous suppurative otitis media – can be considered to be the end result of acute suppurative otitis media in which a permanent perforation of the drum may have developed and the ear drains either continuously or intermittently. The disease may also remain quiescent with a periodically healed drum, only to become active again even with slight environmental changes. The duration of symptoms ranges from 2 months, which for us is the lower limit for truly chronic middle ear disease, up to several years. In a broad sense, all cases of suppurative acute diseases in the middle ear with their complications can be taken into account, since proper handling of the disease at this stage may cure it and prevent the development of chronic suppurative middle ear diseases. Although the treatment of suppurative otitis media with mastoid involvement are dealt with more extensively here, some guide lines for the treatment of the early cases are also offered.

Initially the disease constitutes a bacterial infection in which the common pathogens of the upper respiratory tract, namely Pneumococci, Haemophilus or β-hemolytic Streptococci may be cultured from the ear fluid. The factors which lead to the chronic state are indeed several, e.g. exceptional virulence of the bacteria, lowered resistance of the host, inefficient or too short medication, omission of paracentesis, the presence of large, infected adenoids, problems with nasal ventilation, etc.

Once the suppurative noncholesteatomatous middle ear infection has become chronic itself, the bacterial picture changes. During recurrences of acute upper respiratory tract infections, the Pneumococci and Haemophilus can often be cultured from the ear discharge, but during the chronic stage other bacteria such as Staphylococci, Pseudomonas and Proteus strains are found in culture and especially the latter two can make the disease very resistant to being brought even to a quiescent stage [1].

In order to gather some concrete data on the treatment of the suppurative ears and of its outcome, we have analyzed the records of 51 children hospitalized in this Department because of a chronic suppurative middle ear problem, excluding cases of uncomplicated secretory otitis media and chronic adhesive middle ears. After discussing these cases, we shall take up the subject in its entirety giving an outline of our approach to the management of suppurative otitis media.

Patient Material

On account of the computer filing system in use, it was practical to limit the main study to the period from 1968 to 1976. However, we have counted the number of children's mastoidectomies from the surgery diaries for the years 1966 and 1967 and table I shows an interesting trend. In the years 1966 and 1967, the middle ear ventilation tubes were used only exceptionally and the chronic middle ear problem also involved the mastoid cell system, whereas from 1968 on the tubes were used regularly and early in the treatment of secretory otitis media. At present, our cases of frank suppurative either acute or chronic mastoid disease annually number around 10, while the number of ears with secretory otitis media is ten times larger (in a catchment area of 1.1 million people).

In the series of 51 cases from the period 1968 to 1976, the youngest operated patient was 4 months old and the oldest 15 years, the mean age being 6 years. The distribution into age groups showed a frequency peak during the first 2 years of life, followed by a somewhat smaller rise among the 5- to 6-year-olds.

The duration of symptoms was shorter than 14 days in 25 children and 18 of them were operated on, 7 having a subperiosteal abscess. The disease had lasted 14 days or more in 26 cases (20 over 2 months) and 25 of them were operated upon, 4 with a subperiosteal abscess. Thus, altogether 8 patients were treated conservatively, 7 of whom belonged to the acute and 1 to the chronic group. Practically all patients had received antibiotics prior to surgery.

Table I. Number of children treated in hospital for suppurative middle ear disease

Year	Number of cases
1966	54
1967	46
1968	21
1969	8
1970	15
1971	7
1972	8
1973	8
1974	3
1975	9
1976 (Jan. to June)	3

The leukocyte counts and the sedimentation rates are given in tables II and III. Considering the values normal for the age groups in question, leukocytosis is clearly a less constant phenomenon when evaluating the activity of the infection than is the sedimentation rate, which especially in the acute cases showed a marked increase compared with the normal.

The X-ray findings of the mastoid bone are given in table IV. The constant finding in suppurative acute mastoiditis and in chronic cases is cloudiness of the cell system. The noteworthy feature here is the small or moderate-sized air cell system in the age group of 9–15 years, indicating disturbed pneumatization for a long period of time. Only 2 ears with a large cell system had an acute coalescent mastoiditis.

One sign of the combined effect of the antibiotics used preoperatively, and of the chronicity of the infection, is our finding of only 7 ears with either Pneumococcus, β-hemolytic Streptococcus or Haemophilus infection in this series, while there were 15 ears with Staphylococci and 10 with Pseudomonas strains. Six ears also showed Staphylococci and 4 Pseudomonas strains in the mastoid granulation tissue cultured from the operative specimens. Considering the occasional difficulties in selecting the proper antibiotic, the value of adequate specimens for sensitivity tests cannot be overemphasized [1].

Surgery, when done, should be thorough and the mastoidectomy made complete. If many of the cells are left unopened, the ear does not heal but the infection with granulation tissue formation continues, combined with discharge (fig. 1, 2). Simple mastoidectomy should not be left without supervision at the final stage when done by less experienced surgeons.

Table II. Leukocyte count

	Acute cases		Chronic cases	
	operation	conservative treatment	operation	conservative treatment
< 8,000	6	2	13	–
8–15,000	9	3	10	1
15–20,000	2	1	1	
> 20,000	1	1		
Not studied			1	
Total	18	7	25	1

Table III. Sedimentation rate

SR	Acute cases		Chronic cases		Total
	operation	conservative treatment	operation	conservative treatment	
2– 5			6		6
6–10			7		7
11–20	2	1	7		10
21–30	2				2
31–60	3	2	2	1	8
> 60	11	4	2		17
Not studied			1		1
Total	18	7	25	1	51

Table IV. Preoperative X-ray correlated to age

	Age group			Total
	0–4 years	5–8 years	9–15 years	
Size				
Small + cloudy	5	8	3	16
Moderate + cloudy	9	3	7	19
Large + cloudy	–	–	3	3
No X-ray	9	2	2	13
Total	23	13	15	51

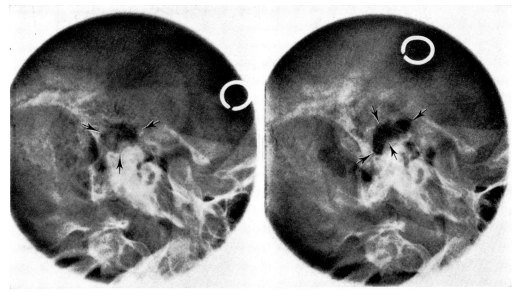

Fig. 1. An example of a poorly performed mastoidectomy in a chronically discharging ear infected with Pseudomonas. The arrows delineate the operation cavity; however, large areas of infected, unopened air cells remain.

Fig. 2. The same ear 1 year after extensive simple mastoidectomy. The arrows now
delineate the area filled with the meatally based musculo-periosteal flap, while the large
posterior cavity, filled with heterograft bone pate, shows signs of ossification without any
depression behind the ear.

In the acute group, 18 ears showed nonperforated tympanic membranes
when admitted to hospital. In all, paracentesis yielded purulent fluid, mostly
under pressure. Seven ears were already discharging due to spontaneous
drum perforation. In the chronic group, there were only 5 nonperforated
drums and paracentesis yielded mucopurulent fluid. 21 ears were discharging,
often for periods exceeding several years.

18 ears of the acute group were subjected to mastoidectomy soon after
admission, including all 7 with subperiosteal abscess. Seven ears were treated
conservatively as the disease after large paracentesis and intensive antibiotic
treatment showed so good an initial response that despite cloudiness of the
cell system early operation was postponed. Of the chronic group, 20 ears
were operated on and only 1 treated conservatively.

Surgery in the acute group consisted of a thorough mastoidectomy
which in some cases was extended into the epitympanic space. In the chronic

Table V. Pre- and postoperative hearing

	Acute		Chronic		Total
	operation	conservative treatment	operation	conservative treatment	
Preoperative (n = 50)					
No audiometry	16	2	10		28
< 20 dB			1		1
20–29 dB	2	3	6		10
30–49 dB		2	6	1	9
> 50 dB			2		2
Postoperative (n = 50)					
No audiometry	8	3	10	1	22
< 20 dB	7	4	4		15
20–29 dB	1		4		4
30–49 dB	2		5		7
> 50 dB			1		2

cases, 16 mastoidectomies were done and 8 extended operations, including myringoplastic repair of the drum defect in 2 ears. One of the latter became adhesive and, in the other, a ventilation tube had to be inserted.

In the acute group, secondary surgery was necessary in 2 ears, 1 of which needed insertion of a ventilation tube because of secretory otitis media and the other tympanotomy and ossicular repair. In chronic ears, further operations were made, including insertion of ventilation tubes in 1 and myringoplasty in 5. In 5 ears, secondary surgery consisted of removal of epitympanic and tympanic granulations and thick mucosa, followed by tympanoplastic repair. The canal wall was kept intact excepting 1 case in which it was reconstructed with a musculo-periosteal flap and cortical bone chips [2].

Results in hearing are given in table V. Due to the young age of many of the patients, audiometric data are not available in all. In older children, hearing is seen to improve satisfactorily postoperatively. In the acute group, 2 patients had hearing between 30 and 50 dB, while there were 5 such ears in the chronic group, and in addition 2 ears with hearing loss exceeding 50 dB. These were all due to tympanic fibrosis and adhesive otitis.

The follow-up data on this series showed that of the operated acute ears 24 (96%) were dry while one continued to drain. In 5 patients, there were later recurrence of acute purulent otitis media which was cured with antibiotic treatment and paracenteses. In the chronic group, the final results showed mobile ear drums in 17 ears (65%). Three showed continuous discharge and 2 had long-term ventilation tubes inserted. Recurrent attacks were later seen and treated in 4 patients.

Case Records

Case 1. This patient was born on August 20, 1969 and at the age of 4 months paracentesis was first performed on both ears. At the age of 1 year, she had urinary infection and was treated in the Pediatric Hospital. She continued to have otitis media attacks several times a year and adenoidectomy was performed at the age of 2 years. During 1972, secretory otitis media developed and tympanostomy tubes were inserted. Rests of the adenoid tissue were removed from the nasal pharynx at this time. The ventilation tubes remained in place for 6 months: the left ear healed, whereas a large central perforation developed in the right ear in 1973. This ear was dry intermittently for some time, but from the end of 1974 it became chronically infected with Pseudomonas and discharge continued without intermission despite continued local treatment.

The patient was admitted for surgery in December, 1975, and the Pseudomonas was sensitive only to colimycin and gentamycin. A thorough mastoidectomy exposing the ossicles in the epitympanum was performed and there was thick secretion together with granulation tissue in the whole mastoid process with distinct areas of bone resorption (fig. 3, 4). The cavity was obliterated with a meatally based musculoperiosteal flap and lyophilized heterograft bone, and the patient was given gentamycin intramuscularly for 9 days. There was some postauricular infection of the soft tissues due to spilling over of irrigation fluid during drilling but this subsided 5 days after surgery. Since no repair of the drum defect was made, colimycin drops were gently pressed through the Eustachian tube twice daily and the patient was discharged on the 10th postoperative day with a dry ear. Despite the large drum defect, hearing in the ear is normal. The ear has now remained asymptomatic for 1 year after surgery.

Comment: Judging from the postoperative course, the use of the proper antibiotic, gentamycin, was essential in the wound healing, and thorough removal of the mastoid pathology enabled the middle ear mucosa to normalize fully. The drum repair will not be made until a few more years have passed without ear problems.

Case 2. This patient was admitted to the Children's Hospital at the age of 4 months on March 21, 1975 with a history of acute ear disease of one week's duration. A postauricular swelling was noted with some injection of the drums. Paracentesis of both ears yielded purulent fluid and treatment with ampicillin was started. Aspiration of the postauricular swelling gave purulent fluid, from which *Klebsiella pneumoniae* and Pneumococci were cultured. A sample taken from the ear canal, curiously enough, yielded Pseudomonas and yellow Staphylococci cultures from the middle ear fluid. The patient was transferred the same day, March 21, to the Ear, Nose, and Throat Hospital where a senior resident performed evacuation of the abscess and an antrotomy the same evening.

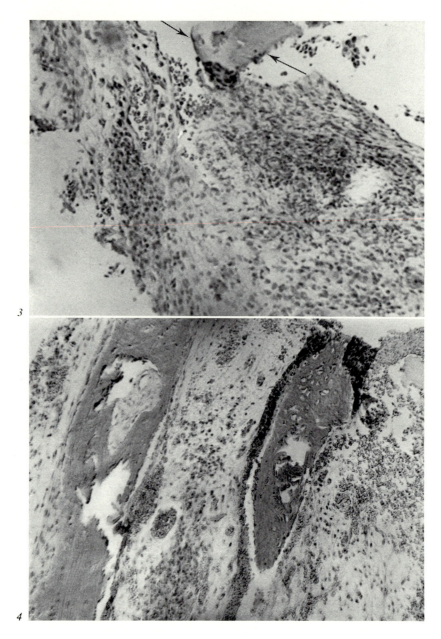

Fig. 3. Infected granulation tissue from mastoid antrum with a small attached bone sequestrum (arrows). × 120.

Fig. 4. Bone biopsy from the area adjoining Trautman's triangle. Much of the bone has been replaced by granulation tissue and the two bone chips show areas of active osteoclastic resorption. × 120.

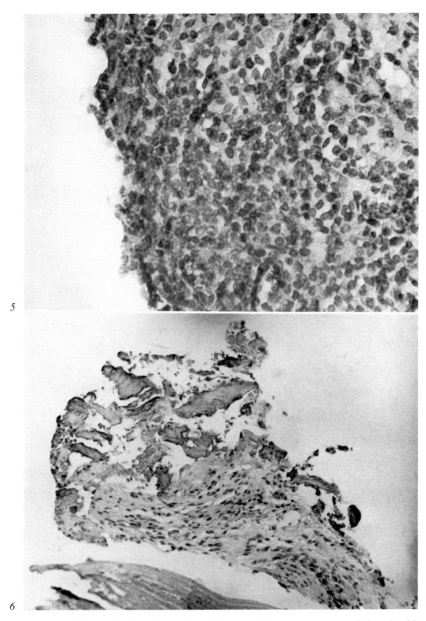

Fig.5. Fresh granulation tissue from the mastoid antrotomy area, infected with Pseudomonas. × 240.

Fig.6. Sequestered dead bone chips and granulation tissue from the central area of the mastoid. × 72.

The left ear continued to drain profusely from the postauricular incision with a pure growth of Pseudomonas, sensitive only to gentamycin and colimycin. At this time, senior staff was consulted and the patient prepared for thorough extended mastoidectomy. The mastoid bone was full of granulation tissue and osteomyelitic-looking bone (fig. 5, 6), and Pseudomonas was cultured from specimens taken during surgery. The cavity was obliterated and the ear healed under gentamycin systemic treatment in 10 days.

One month later, the child had symptoms of common cold and paracentesis of both ears yielded mucoid secretion. The left ear normalized in 1 month, but repeated paracenteses had to be performed for 2 months before fluid ceased to form on the right. Two months later, the patient again had coryza and both ears contained purulent fluid with Haemophilus infection. Secretory process continued and on September 9, 1975, adenotomy was performed with insertion of ventilation tubes in both ears. At home, both ears started discharging and the patient was admitted again. The cytotoxic leukocyte test [3] was by now fully worked out in our laboratory and the patient proved to have a 3+ reaction to milk, 2+ to wheat and 1+ to tomatoes. These were all removed from the diet and since October 1975 the patient has been symptom-free.

Comment: This very infection-prone child developed acute mastoiditis, for which initial antrotomy was totally insufficient. Only after thorough mastoidectomy was the disease brought under control. However, the child remained infection-prone and the picture of secretory otitis media developed, to be interrupted only with acute discharge episodes. Only with the aid of the cytotoxic leukocyte test was the food allergy (most serious milk) discovered and dietary control brought an end to the year-long history of recurrent upper respiratory infections.

Management of Suppurative Middle Ear Disease

1. The Acute Stage

Proper management of the initial disease is of crucial importance since in our experience ears myringomized the first day and given proper antibiotic treatment almost never develop chronic changes. At present, there is a controversy whether a paracentesis should be made or not and some statistics claim that it is not necessary. One of us (T.P.) observed one study in Finland closely as long as 25 years ago [4] and arbitrary selection of cases had to be discontinued and paracentesis performed because earache continued and disease spread in several cases, initially falling into the group to be treated without paracentesis. In our experience, paracentesis can be omitted in those ears in which the hearing is still good and the drum is in normal position and mobile, and a course of V-penicillin given for 10 days. If there is any doubt of Haemophilus infection, the drug initially chosen should be either erythromycin, ampicillin or amoxicillin. If symptoms continue in the form of earache or hearing deteriorates, paracentesis should be made.

When the first attack of purulent otitis media occurs, the patient's adenoid status should be evaluated. This is even more important if a recurrence occurs. In our experience, early removal of the adenoids prevents many of the possible future recurrences, and the development of chronic ear disease. Removal at a late stage, when the secretory otitis media type of a disease has already developed, does not give the same help as does an early operation. However, we stress that surgery should be done under proper general anesthesia and final removal of the adenoid rests around the choanae be made with angulated forceps with the help of a laryngeal mirror.

If acute mastoiditis with a subperiosteal abscess develops, thorough simple mastoidectomy should be performed immediately and a large paracentesis opening made to guarantee the free flow of pus away from the middle ear. At this stage, changes in the mucosa are caused by reversible edema and the inserting of drainage tubes, or mucous membrane removal, is not indicated.

Similar treatment should be adopted if the roentgen examination reveals a coalescent mastoiditis without an abscess. However, cases with only cloudiness in the cell system can in some cases be observed for a few days, and if paracentesis and effective antibiotic treatment seem to halt the disease, mastoidectomy may become unnecessary. When in doubt, we favor the more radical method. Every case of purulent otitis media should be checked in 10–14 days. If there is still some disease going on, more active treatment should be adopted.

2. Subacute and Subchronic Stage

This period extends from 2 weeks to 2 months, the first 3 weeks belonging to the subacute and the latter 3 to the subchronic stage. A new paracentesis in the subacute stage is mandatory if the drum has healed, or the ear shows a scant discharge with retention in the middle ear. If the treatment has begun with V-penicillin, this should be changed into amoxicillin or erythromycin as it is almost certain that Haemophilus infection has been the initial cause. After the visit, we advise a weekly check of the ear, have the bacterial sensitivity tests made, and do the mastoid X-ray examination.

If the ear has not healed during the second treatment period, we advise the patient to be admitted to hospital for further treatment. This generally leads to adenoid surgery and insertion of the ventilation tubes, possibly combined with simple mastoidectomy. Studies of the serum immunoglobulin, including IgE, has only in exceptional cases been found to have any decisive importance in treatment. Lack of iron in our series has not been evident

either, and only in 2 cases has the hemoglobin value been under 10 g. However, at this stage, or in children with recurrent infection, the cytotoxic
leukocyte test should be made since removal of an offending food may put
an end to the whole infection cycle.

3. Chronic Stage

At this stage, the initial attack of otitis media may have proceeded in
various directions. Chronical discharge generally indicates definite pathology
on one or both sides of the middle ear, namely in the mastoid cell system
and/or in the adenoid – post nasal – sinus area. The development of typical
secretory otitis media is at present one of the largest groups but will be dealt
with here only when combined with mastoid infection. Finally, at this stage
there are the established chronic ears with adhesive otitis media giving symptoms only in the form of severe hearing loss.

The chronically or periodically discharging ears show a permanent drum
defect in the pars tensa, small mastoid cell systems with cloudiness or
sclerosis. A polypoid, thick middle ear mucosa may be seen through the
perforation. Adenoid surgery has generally been made and the blood values
are within normal limits. Bacterial sensitivity tests are now mandatory and
daily irrigation with saline combined with local treatment with ear drops
should first be employed during the conservative treatment. We try to select
the ear drops according to the sensitivity tests but avoid the ototoxic antibiotics locally. If not done earlier, the leukocyte cytotoxic test should be
made (case 2).

We have generally limited the surgery in children to thorough mastoidectomy, combined either with removal of polypoid mucosa via the ear
canal through the perforation, or in healed drums, with insertion of the
ventilation tubes. Systemic antibiotic treatment should be started a day
before surgery; during surgery, we thoroughly irrigate the ear alternatively
with 3% hydrogen perioxide solution and physiological saline. It would be
too optimistic to think that surgery alone with limited access to middle ear
in children would cure, for example, a longstanding Pseudomonas infection.

We do not advocate tympanoplastic repair in children's ear, but leave the
perforation open and repair it 1 year later, if the middle ear has remained
dry and healed well. A two-stage surgery seems advisable to us, since in discharging ears the middle ear mucosa possesses the secretory properties
characteristic of secretory otitis media [5], and to repair the perforation
would deprive the ear of the necessary ventilation from the ear canal at this
stage. Furthermore, surgical intervention in the middle ear would add many

new raw surfaces from which new connective tissue would start to grow and, due to the lack of good Eustachian tube function, would eventually lead to totally adhesive middle ear.

Our present surgical method, not used throughout the series, however, due to the change of Department Head in 1974, includes closing of the epitympanic antral, and the possibly opened facial recess area with the meatally based musculoperiosteal flap. This was primarily made to prevent any future infection from spreading into the mastoid space again [6]. At present, we consider cavity obliteration to be even more important from the viewpoint that it prevents the development of posterior drum quadrant invagination, due to possible underpressure, towards the antrum, and prevents a subsequent development of cholesteatoma. If the Eustachian tube begins to function normally, the total middle ear area provides an air volume entirely sufficient to guarantee an absolutely normal function. Definite proof that mastoid air space is not necessary for normal middle ear function are the cases with hereditary absence of mastoid air cells as well as the fenestrated ears with otosclerosis in which an effective and many times very large cell system was surgically removed without any harmful effect upon the middle ear aeration.

Finally, it is the surgeon's duty to keep the operated cases under continuous surveillance and not to dismiss them a few weeks after surgery. Yearly check-ups should be done during the healed stage until the child is grown up and, during each visit, evaluation of the ear should be made not only by eye but also by audiometry and tympanometry. Adequate steps can then be taken to remedy any possible new activity of the ear disease.

References

1   PALVA, T.: Bacterial analyses in chronic otitis media. ORL Digest 33: 19–26 (1971).
2   PALVA, T.: Obliterative technique in mastoid obliteration. Acta oto-lar. 75: 289–290 (1973).
3   BRYAN, W.T.K. and BRYAN, M.P.: Cytotoxic reactions in the diagnosis of food allergy. Otolaryng. Clin. N. Am. 4: 523–534 (1971).
4   HEIKKILÄ, S. und PELTONEN, T: Über die Mittelohrentzündungen der Kinder. Mschr. Kinderheilk. 104: 463–466 (1956).
5   KARMA, P. and PALVA, T.: Middle ear epithelium in chronic ear disease. Acta oto-lar. 75: 271–272 (1973).
6   PALVA, T.: Mastoiditis in children. Laryngoscope 72: 353–360 (1962).

T. PALVA, MD, Department of Otolaryngology, University of Helsinki, Helsinki (Finland)

Adv. Oto-Rhino-Laryng., vol. 23, pp. 58–64 (Karger, Basel 1978)

Management of Cholesteatoma in Children

JAMES L. SHEEHY

The Otologic Medical Group, Inc. and
The Ear Research Institute, Los Angeles, Calif.

Few would doubt the need for surgery in cases of cholesteatoma. But is there a difference in management of the disease in children? Are complications of the disease different in children? Should the surgical technique of mastoidectomy be different in children than in adults? What part does Eustachian tube function play in the decision regarding surgery? Do the results of reconstructive middle ear and mastoid surgery in children differ from those in adults?

In the following pages, I will give you answers to these questions based on our experience at the Otologic Medical Group, Inc., Los Angeles.

Patient Population

We reviewed the charts of 1,024 patients operated upon for cholesteatoma over a 10-year period ending in December, 1974. All were primary operations in which the cholesteatoma involved, but was not limited to, the epitympanum or mastoid.

181 of these operations (18 %) were performed on individuals under 16 years of age. The youngest was 4 and there were 33 cases between ages 4 and 6. From this point forward, I will refer to this group (under 16) as children and the remainder as adults.

Complications of the Disease

A labyrinthine fistula, facial weakness, total sensori-neural impairment, meningeal complication or a combination of these complications was present in 11 % of these cholesteatoma cases [1].

A labyrinthine fistula was by far the most common complication (10 %), but was present in only 4 % of the children.

Facial nerve weakness or total loss of hearing occurred infrequently (1 %) and was less frequent in the children (no total sensorineurals and only one facial weakness).

There were only three instances of meningeal complications (one meningitis and two chronic subdural abscesses) and none of these occurred in the children. We suspect that this does not represent a true picture of meningeal complications and could be explained by the necessity of admitting all patients with meningitis of unexplained origin in Los Angeles to the County Communicable Disease Facility.

When these four complications were evaluated both in regard to age of the patient and duration of the disease in various age groups, it became apparent that complications of the disease were for the most part related to duration of disease. In those 348 patients whose disease had been apparent for 20 years or more, the incidence of complication was 19 %. In those whose disease was thought to have existed less than 10 years (522), the incidence was 7 %.

Surgical Technique

Our surgical techniques for the management of aural cholesteatoma have been published and there is little need to restate them [2, 3]. Cholesteatoma involving the mastoid may be managed by the classical radical or modified radical mastoidectomy (exteriorization procedure) or by mastoidectomy combined with tympanoplasty (reconstructive procedure).

Tympanoplasty with mastoidectomy is an operation performed to eradicate disease in the middle ear and mastoid and to reconstruct the hearing mechanism, with or without tympanic membrane grafting [4]. It may involve creation of an open mastoid cavity (cavity technique), creation of a cavity followed by obliteration with soft tissue or bone (obliteration technique) or the closed technique, the intact canal wall procedure, in which normal anatomical contours of the ear canals are not significantly modified. We prefer the intact canal wall procedure whenever possible because of its obvious advantages to the patient: The healed ear may be treated normally, with minimal postoperative care required.

The majority of our cases were managed by the intact canal wall procedure (table I) and there were few differences in the management of children

Table I. Chronic otitis media with cholesteatoma: operative procedure performed (n = 1,024).

Procedure	Incidence, %
Tympanoplasty	97.6
Intact canal wall (88.1%)	
Obliteration (6.9%)	
Cavity remains (2.6%)	
Modified Radical or Radical	2.4

Table II. Tympanoplasty with mastoidectomy for cholesteatoma: reason for staging the operation related to age of patient

	All cases (n = 996)	Age of patient, years		
		4–6 (n = 32)	7–15 (n = 145)	16+ (n = 819)
Operation staged, %	39	68	46	36
Reason for staging:				
Residual disease involved in decision for staging, %	50	68	71	44
Residual disease *only* reason for staging, %	12	9	14	10

Table III. Tympanoplasty with mastoidectomy for cholesteatoma: incidence of residual disease in planned second-stage operation

	Age of patient, years	
	4–15 (n = 82)	16 or older (n = 221)
Incidence of residual disease, %	51	30
Residual found in both middle ear and epitympanum or mastoid, %	13	5
Residual limited to middle ear, %	27	16
Residual limited to epitympanum or mastoid, %	11	9

and adults. 90 % of the operations in children were intact canal wall procedure. A radical or modified radical mastoidectomy was performed in 1 % of
the children as opposed to 2 ½ % of the adults.

The major arguments in regard to tympanoplasty with mastoidectomy
involve the matter of safety of a closed technique as opposed to an open
technique. Arguments in this regard differ little whether one is talking about
children or adults; it is only a matter of degree. Some who feel that closed
techniques are acceptable in adults do not feel they are acceptable in children
due to the more 'malignant' nature of cholesteatoma in children and the
possibility of residual disease. Because of this concern, we are more likely
to perform surgery in two stages in children.

Staging the Operation

The concept of performing surgery for cholesteatoma as a planned two-
stage operation was first introduced by RAMBO in 1961 and further clarified
by TABB [5].

It was not until the mid 1960s, however, that we began staging cholesteatoma surgery in a systematic way. In recent years, we have been staging
50 % of our tympanoplasty with mastoidectomy cases and have recently
reported the indications and results [5].

Planned staging of the operation may be indicated for one or both of
two reasons: to obtain a better hearing result or to obtain an ear free of
both residual and recurrent cholesteatoma. The decision is made at the time
of surgery and is based on a consideration of the mucosal and ossicular
problem encountered and the possibility of residual disease. Our main concern here is the matter of residual disease: cholesteatoma left behind by the
surgeon.

The possibility (or probability?) of leaving cholesteatoma in the ear, and
the potential seriousness of this, is the major point of argument in regard to
the open versus the closed operation. We believe that it is preferable not to
create a permanently exteriorized mastoid cavity and to reexplore selected
cases for residual disease.

The percentage of our cholesteatoma cases managed by the intact canal
wall technique is the same in children and in adults. We are more likely to
reexplore the ear in children and the reason for this is our concern in regard
to residual disease (table II).

Table III shows the location and incidence of residual disease at the time of the planned second-stage operation. Residual disease was almost twice as common in the children, but the location of this residual disease was similar in the two groups. In looking at this high incidence of residual disease, you must remember that the figures refer to the findings in planned second-stage procedures, and that the possibility of this residual disease was often the primary reason for reexploring the ear. It does point out, however, the need for a high index of suspicion!

In both children and adults, residual disease was found in the epitympanum or mastoid (and usually this was the epitympanum) less frequently than in the middle ear. In adults, a middle ear residuum was found in 21 % as apposed to 14 % in the epitympanum. In children, a middle ear residuum was found in 40 % as apposed to 24 % in the epitympanum.

Eustachian Tube Function

Some place great emphasis on evaluation of Eustachian tube function prior to reconstruction surgery in cases of chronic otitis media, and this is especially true in the case of children.

We no longer test Eustachian tube function routinely prior to tympanoplasty. Although it was originally stated that tympanoplasty could not be performed in the face of Eustachian tube blockage, we soon learned that the majority of patients manifesting poor function preoperatively maintained good function postoperatively [6]. Conclusion: The best treatment for the Eustachian tube in chronic otitis media is to operate upon the ear and rid it of disease.

It was then stated that the operation would not be successful if the Eustachian tube were malfunctioning. We found that in the small percentage of cholesteatoma cases with persistent tubal malfunction postoperatively, we could ventilate the ear transtympanically and maintain satisfactory hearing [7].

The subject of Eustachian tube function tests in cases of cholesteatoma is really academic. An ear with cholesteatoma usually does not have a perforation open to the Eustachian tube, and when it does there is usually so much inflammatory change in the mucosa that Eustachian tube blockage would be anticipated.

Persistent postoperative serous otitis media occurred in only 4 % of the tympanoplasty cases. The incidence was highest in the 6 and under age group (2/33) and lowest in the 7- to 15-year age group (1/148).

Results of Surgery

I have already commented upon the fact that we perform a planned two-stage operation in over half of our children with cholesteatoma (table II). The incidence of residual disease in these planned revisions is 51 % (table III).

The fascia graft take rate in the 996 tympanoplasty cases was the same in children as in adults: 97 %. 2 % of the cases having a successful result at 6 months have later developed tympanic membrane perforation.

Persistent postoperative serous otitis was infrequent (4 %), but occurred slightly more frequently in those between the ages of 4 and 6 (2/33).

We have detected no difference in the hearing results between the adults and the children. Generally speaking, the children undergoing tympanomastoid surgery heal faster and have fewer problems than the adults. Most of us would prefer to limit our otologic surgery to children were this possible.

Conclusions

(1) Complications of cholesteatoma are less common in the younger age group due primarily to the shorter duration of the disease.

(2) The surgical techniques employed in the management of cholesteatoma in children are the same as in adults.

(3) Those who use the intact canal wall technique in the management of aural cholesteatoma, as we do, should seriously consider reexploration of the mastoid and middle ear in most of their cases. Residual cholesteatoma is more frequently found in the middle ear.

(4) Measurement of Eustachian tube function plays no part in the evaluation for surgery in cases of cholesteatoma. The incidence of persistent postoperative serous otitis media is low.

(5) There has been no detectable difference in the results of tympanoplasty with mastoidectomy for cholesteatoma when comparing children with adults.

References

1   SHEEHY, J.L.; BRACKMANN, D.E., and GRAHAM, M.D.: Complications of cholesteatoma: A report of 1024 cases. 1st Int. Conf. Cholesteatoma, Iowa City 1976.
2   SHEEHY, J.L. and PATTERSON, M.D.: Intact canal wall tympanoplasty with mastoidectomy. Laryngoscope 77: 1502 (1967).

3   SHEEHY, J.L.: Surgery of chronic otitis media; in Otolaryngology, vol.2, chap.10
     (Harper & Row, Hagerstown 1972).
4   Committee on Conservation of Hearing of the American Academy of Ophthalmology
     and Otolaryngology: Standard classification for Surgery of chronic ear infection.
     Archs Otolar. *81:* 204 (1965).
5   SHEEHY, J.L. and CRABTREE, J.A.: Tympanoplasty: staging the operation. Laryngo-
     scope *83:* 1594 (1973).
6   HOUSE, W.F. and SHEEHY, J.L.: Functional restoration in tympanoplasty. Archs
     Otolar. *78:* 304 (1963).
7   SHEEHY, J.L.: Collar button tube chronic serous otitis. Trans.Am.Acad.Ophthal.
     Oto-lar. *68:* 888 (1964).

J.L.SHEEY, MD, The Otologic Medical Group, Inc. and The Ear Research Institute,
Los Angeles, Calif. (USA)

Adv. Oto-Rhino-Laryng., vol. 23, pp. 65–72 (Karger, Basel 1978)

Choanal Atresia

BRUCE BENJAMIN

Sydney University, Sydney

Anterior choanal atresia is extremely rare and the term choanal atresia is usually taken to mean congenital posterior choanal atresia due to a bony obstruction (occasionally partly membranous) of the posterior end of the nasal cavity. The atresia may be bilateral, when it presents as an acute, life-threatening respiratory obstruction in the newborn baby or it may be unilateral when it is usually detected weeks, months or even many years after birth.

The anomaly was first recorded by ROEDERER [5] in 1755 and the first transnasal perforation was by EMMERT [3] in 1851.

The diagnosis is made more often in the neonatal period with increasing awareness of the condition amongst pediatricians, obstetricians and otolaryngologists. In many nurseries, it is part of the routine physical examination of a newborn baby to pass catheters through each nasal cavity. The increased number of babies surviving with this condition is, to some extent, a result of earlier and better management of the associated congenital anomalies which are commonly present. Associated congenital anomalies of minor or major degree have been variously reported in from 30 to 50 % of patients [2, 4, 5], but there is no consistent association with any particular anomaly or set of anomalies.

The exact incidence of the condition is not known but it is not uncommon in large pediatric hospitals. It is commoner in females and unilateral atresia is predominantly right-sided [5].

The etiology of choanal atresia is not known. A familial tendency has been quoted by several authors [5, 10] but is unusual.

During the sixth week of fetal life, the bucconasal membrane normally

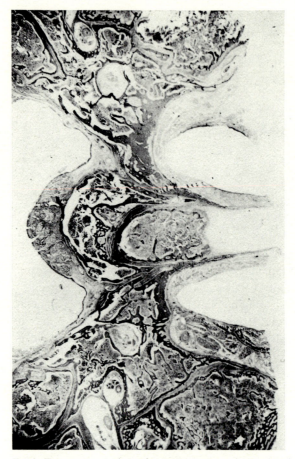

Fig.1. Transverse section of postmortem specimen showing site of bony atresia anterior to the posterior end of the nasal septum.

ruptures to connect the primitive nasal cavities with the pharynx [4, 5, 8]. Despite a difference of opinion amongst embryologists to satisfactorily explain the abnormality, the presence of membranous atresia may be accounted for by failure of the bucconasal membrane to rupture. This is not a satisfactory explanation for the presence of bony atresia although it has been postulated that persistent islands of mesoderm later organize into bone.

The atresia is usually some millimeters anterior to the exact plane of the posterior choanae themselves (fig. 1).

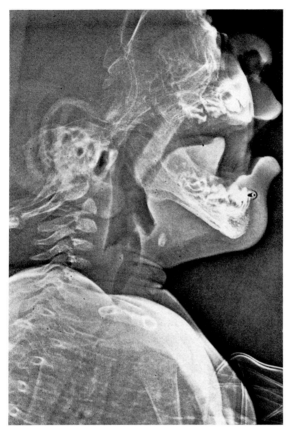

Fig. 2. Lateral xeroradiogram showing air filling the postnasal space, but no air in the nasal cavitiy, in a patient with bilateral choanal atresia.

Diagnosis

Complete obstruction of the nasal airways at birth produces acute respiratory embarassment. The baby makes vigorous respiratory efforts with marked chest retraction, impaired pulmonary ventilation, progressive cyanosis, bradycardia as hypoxia increases and possibly death from asphyxia if prompt and appropriate treatment is not instituted. However, if the infant cries and takes a deep breath through the mouth, the airway obstruction is momentarily relieved. The high larynx of the neonate with the epiglottis adjacent to the soft palate, the powerful naso-respiratory reflex and the fact that the newborn child will not normally breathe through his mouth, even when there is nasal obstruction, means impending suffocation unless the seriousness of the nasal obstruction is recognized and emergency measures are taken.

Patency of each side of the nose may be tested simply with a wisp of cotton wool or by looking for frosting on a mirror or a silvered surface. A diagnosis of nasal obstruction may be confirmed by failure to pass a catheter or probe through the nose into the pharynx, by failure of methylene blue instilled into the nose to appear in the pharynx, by failure to gently blow air through the nasal cavity with a Politzer bag or by auscultation at the anterior nares. A lateral xeroradiogram may support the diagnosis (fig. 2).

It is possible, but unnecessary, to radiologically confirm posterior nasal obstruction by installation of contrast material into the nasal cavity after suction clearance of excessive mucus and application of a suitable decongestant.

Other causes of serious nasal obstruction in a neonate include trauma to the nose or nasal septum, hypertrophy of the nasal turbinates, encephalocele, dermoid, hamartoma, etc.

A final certain diagnosis and differentiation from rarer causes of nasal or postnasal obstruction may be made under general anesthetic with examination of the nasal cavity and nasopharynx transnasally and behind the palate with mirrors and angled telescopes (fig. 3) [4]. This confirmation is essential before any attempt at surgical correction is made.

Bilateral choanal atresia therefore always produces symptoms in the neonatal period, but it is curious that the degree of respiratory obstruction and cyanosis varies from one patient to another and even in the same patient from time to time. Besides the severe respiratory obstruction, there is feeding difficulty because of inability to co-ordinate swallowing and breathing so that aspiration pneumonia may occur with accompanying changes on the chest X-ray.

Unilateral posterior choanal atresia is associated with a persistent, thick, mucoid discharge, but does not cause noticeable respiratory distress unless the normally patent nasal cavity becomes congested or blocked in the young baby for some unrelated reason (e.g. an upper respiratory tract infection). There is then real respiratory distress and difficulty with feeding. Thus, unilateral atresia is often undiagnosed in the neonatal period and may in fact be overlooked until the patient is some months or even some years old. Surgical correction may be delayed and is usually advisable before the child commences school.

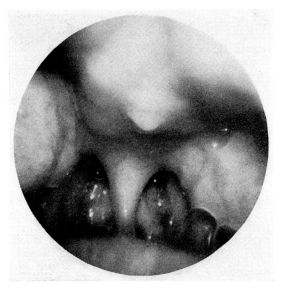

Fig. 3. Photograph taken with a 120° telescope behind the palate of a neonate.

Management

Having recognized the nature of the neonatal respiratory emergency, an adequate oral airway must be provided promptly. This may be achieved by use of the McGovern nipple [7], or of a Guedel oral airway [4], by introduction of a per-oral endotracheal tube, or by use of an oro-esophageal tube.

Recently at the Royal Alexandra Hospital for Children, Sydney, we have provided a satisfactory artificial airway using an oro-esophageal tube (fig. 4, 5). The technique is simple, the equipment is readily available in every obstetric ward or nursery and any medical or nursing attendant can apply the method. Its use as an emergency procedure is apparently free from any serious complications. A wide diameter plastic tube (approximately 16 French gauge) is passed through the mouth into the mid-esophagus. This maintains a patent oro-pharyngeal airway by holding the tongue forward, keeping the mouth open and providing a roughly triangular airway each side of the tube. A fine (5 French gauge) feeding tube is passed through the wider tube into the stomach for feeding purposes and to vent the stomach. The larger tube is firmly fixed to the child's face. The smaller tube is secured as

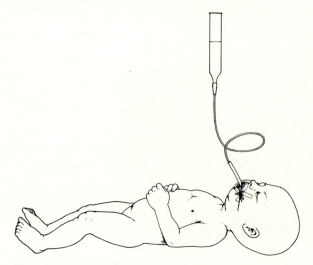

Fig. 4. Oro-esophageal intubation.

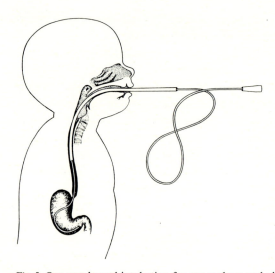

Fig. 5. Oro-esophageal intubation for nasopahryngeal obstruction in the neonate.

it passes out the proximal end of the larger tube. This technique may be used for several weeks or more in bilateral choanal atresia.

It is worth noting that this simple technique may be used also in patients with obstruction of the pharyngeal airway due to micrognathia and retro-position of the tongue, where simpler forms of management are ineffective.

It is our current approach to use such an oro-esophageal tube in bilateral choanal atresia for several weeks until the child satisfactorily learns mouth breathing, is feeding well and is gaining weight. He is then discharged from hospital, reviewed regularly and a transnasal operation is performed on one side at about 12 months of age. The second side is similarly operated at between 2 and 4 years of age with dilatation or revision of the first side where necessary. Transpalatal surgery is reserved for unsatisfactory results using this technique. This conservative surgical approach cannot be applied to all cases, but it is felt that surgical morbidity or mortality in the neonatal period will be minimized and a more satisfactory long-term result achieved.

Tracheotomy should have no place in the management of an otherwise uncomplicated bilateral choanal atresia.

Many surgical procedures have been advocated either in the neonatal period or delayed until some months or even years later. Most babies achieve the ability to breathe through their mouth and feed adequately in from 3 to 8 weeks. If a satisfactory airway and good nutrition can be maintained during this period, surgical correction can be delayed until a more suitable and convenient age.

Surgical treatments advocated in the neonatal period include electro-coagulation of the atretic plate [6], transnasal puncture of the partition [1] with dilatation and enlargement of the bony apperture using curettes or bone biting forceps, commonly followed by placement of a plastic tube through the nasal cavity for some days or weeks. The risk of perforation into the spinal canal is small but significant. After early intranasal operation, further dilatations or later revision operations may be necessary for fibrous annular scar tissue or even bony regrowth.

It has become popular recently to advocate definitive treatment by transpalatal operation [2, 5, 9] in the newborn period. Various incisions in the palate are described, the soft palate is detached from the edge of the hard palate preserving the superior mucosal layer, and the posterior edge of the hard palate is removed together with the posterior part of the nasal septum with an attempt to preserve mucosal flaps once the atresia has been satisfactorily dealt with surgically. After positioning of the mucoperiosteal flaps, plastic tubes are usually left in the nasal cavity on each side for up to a week.

The many approaches to management and surgical correction attest to the difficulties which have been encountered. No obviously superior results are available to dictate a uniformly successful approach.

References

1 BEINFIELD, H. H.: Bilateral choanal atresia in the newborn. Archs Otolar. *73:* 659–661 (1961).
2 CHERRY, J. and BORDLEY, J.: Surgical correction of choanal atresia. Ann. Otol. Rhinol. Lar. *75:* 911–920 (1966).
3 EMMERT, C. F.: Lehrbuch der Chirurgie (Dann, Stuttgart 1853).
4 FEARON, B. and DICKSON, J.: Bilateral choanal atresia in the newborn. Plan of action. Laryngoscope *78:* 1487–1499 (1968).
5 FLAKE, C. G. and FERGUSON, C. F.: Congenital choanal atresia in infants and children. Ann. Otol. Rhinol. Lar. *73:* 458–473 (1964).
6 HERRMANN, I. F. and KLEIN, P. P.: Electrocoagulation in the treatment of the choanal atresia in the newborn. J. Lar. Otol. *84:* 1257–1260 (1970).
7 MCGOVERN, F. H.: Bilateral choanal atresia in the newborn. A new method of medical management. Laryngoscope *71:* 480–483 (1961).
8 MCKIBBEN, B. G.: Congenital atresia of the nasal choanae. Laryngoscope *67:* 731–755 (1957).
9 RUDDY, L. W.: A transpalatine operation for congenital atresia of the choanae in the small child or infant. Archs Otolar. *41:* 432–438 (1945).
10 WILKERSON, W. W., jr. and CAYME, L. F.: Congenital choanal occlusion. Trans. Am. Acad. Ophthal. Oto-lar. *52:* 234–246 (1948).

B. BENJAMIN, OBE, MB, BS, DLO, F.R.A.C.S., Lecturer in Diseases of the Ear, Nose and Throat, Sydney University, *Sydney* (Australia)

Adv. Oto-Rhino-Laryng., vol. 23, pp. 73–86 (Karger, Basel 1978)

Nasopharyngoscopy and Sinoscopy in Children

Basharat Jazbi

Department of Otorhinolaryngology, University of Missouri, Kansas City, School of Medicine, The Children's Mercy Hospital, Kansas City, Mo.

With 1 colour plate

Introduction

Nasopharyngoscopy and sinoscopy are not new techniques, however, their revival and application in its refined form is relatively recent. The idea evolved in 1902 by Hirschmann and later by Reichert who realized that a cystoscope could be used in the examination and diagnosis of the diseases of the maxillary sinus. However, they did not succeed in popularizing this technique. It fell out of vogue rather rapidly and remained dormant for several years [4, 6]. The concept and the technique was basically the same as practiced now. However, in the beginning both Hirschmann and Reichert used sinoscopy by drilling a hole in the canine fossa or through a dental alveolus as the route of choice. But in 1922, Speilberg modified the method by using a straight trocar and entering the maxillary sinus through the nose under the inferior turbinate. Although this method was relatively easy, it did not catch on for nearly half a century. However, it was occasionally practiced at a few centers by otolaryngologists and some dental surgeons as described by Bethmann in 1953. In the last two decades this technique has been, with some modifications, revived and practiced in Germany and other European countries. However, the introduction of cold fiberoptic lights and Hopkins optic telescopes have revolutionized this technique as it has done in other areas of endoscopy.

Whether it is nasopharynx or the maxillary sinuses, we are confronted with hidden, dark cavities and more often than not it is a blind procedure [8]. In the nasopharynx, the method of examination is indirect examination or digital palpation. In the maxillary sinuses the diagnosis is generally made either by aspiration of fluid from the antrum or by X-ray examination,

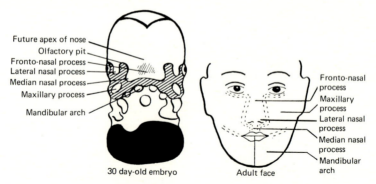

Fig. 1. Development of nose. Reproduced from SIMPSON *et al.* [20].

which, as we all know is not always reliable. In recent years, microsurgery of the nose has been introduced in order to obtain a better view and proper access to the later nasal wall structures [9, 10].

Embryology

The paranasal sinuses develop as evaginations from the nasal chambers. The development begins in fetal life and early childhood and continues to expand in size and shape until adolescence [2, 8]. The maxillary sinus is the first one to develop and like others does so as an evagination in the middle meatus of the embryo of 80–90 days of fetal life. Nasal development is obvious in a 30-day embryo [15, 20] (fig. 1). The sinus cavity continues to expand and at birth it measures approximately $2 \times 2 \times 1$ cm and lies below the eye high in the maxilla [2, 17, 19] (fig. 2). As the skull growth and dentition occurs, it expands in size from above downwards occupying the space of the erupted teeth in the alveolus. By the age of about 11, the sinus expands considerably and its lowermost portion is at the level of the floor of the nose [15, 18]. Further development occurs slowly as secondary dentition proceeds, and is complete between the age of 15–18 years. The maxillary sinuses are generally tubular in infants, oval in childhood and pyramidal in shape in adults [2, 18, 20] (fig. 3). In an adult, the floor of the maxillary sinus is even at a lower level than the floor of the nose [2, 8, 14].

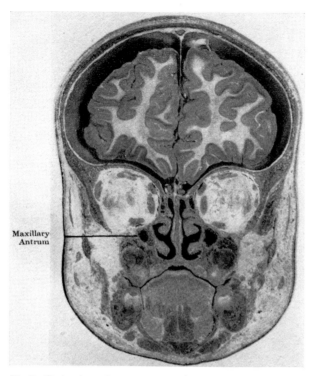

Fig. 2. Coronal section, age approximately 1 year, showing the position of the maxillary sinus. Reproduced from WILSON [18].

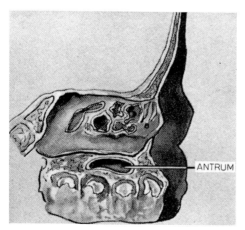

Fig. 3. Diagrammatic representation showing tubular antrum in infants. Reproduced from WILSON [18].

Inflammations

Although paranasal sinus disease in childhood is not very common, contrary to general belief that it is very unlikely to develop before the age of 2–3 years, sinusitis is clinically present at a very early age. However, the size of the paranasal sinus cavity in a child is relatively smaller in contrast to the size of the ostium so that retention of secretions does not occur. Thus, while a viral rhinitis might extend to the antrum and destroy the cilia of the membrane, the mucus in the cavity is easily expelled due to a relatively large ostium as compared to the size of the maxillary cavity and the secretions it can hold [8, 14, 19]. Some of the causative factors are unilateral choanal atresia, foreign body in the nose, allergy, trauma (facial fracture), swimming, deviated nasal septum, nasal polyps, cystic fibrosis, viral infections and immune deficiency [5, 7, 18, 20].

Maxillary Sinus

The ostium is the site of the original evagination of the sinus from the nasal chamber. Because the sinuses are outgrowths of the nasal chamber, their mucus membrane is ciliated columnar epithelium which is similar to that of nasal cavity. Differences lie in the sparsity of cilia and mucus glands as the membrane is thinner and the columnar cells smaller in height than the ones found elsewhere in the nasal mucosa [2, 12, 14, 17].

The sinus becomes infected because of its dependent position in relation to the ostium of the sinus, which lies at a more superior position so that secretions are retained within the lumen and must be swept towards the ostium by the cilia [2, 14, 17]. Thus the sinus infection is more apt to occur in the older child in the pre-teen and teen years (fig. 4). Although as stated before, it is encountered in early childhood. The usual causative bacterial agents are α- and β-streptococcus, diplococcus, *Stapylococcus aureus*, *Haemophilus influenzae* and *Escherichia coli*.

Pain may be appreciated in the teeth or the face of the maxilla and may be referred even to the forehead above the eye, or laterally in the temple [8, 14]. The patient often blows purulent material from the nose and some of it may be seen cascading into the pharynx on nasopharyngoscopy using a fiberoptic telescope [7, 8, 19]. Other associated signs are nasal obstruction, purulent discharge, cough and sneezing, epistaxis, otitis media, leukocytosis, pyrexia, and pharyngitis and lymphangitis. However, for obvious reasons

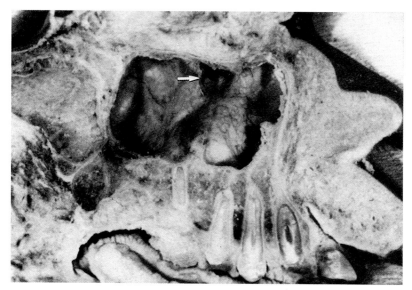

Fig.4. Location and size of natural ostium. Reproduced from RITTER [14].

diagnosis in infants is more difficult than in older children. Treatment of the acute phase should be with the appropriate antibiotics selected on the basis of the knowledge that this is mostly a gram-positive infection.

When chronic infection occurs, the first step in its management is to remove the retained secretions by irrigation [14, 19]. Some surgeons prefer inserting the trocar into the cavity via an approach under the upper lip after a radiographic determination of the size of the maxillary sinus [4, 8, 19]. Once within the cavity the obturator of the cannula is withdrawn and aspiration is used to detect either air or mucopurulent debris. Irrigation can then proceed in a safe manner [1, 8]. However, in children over the age of 5, sinoscopy can be done and is preferred at our hospital.

Sinoscopy

Instruments

The instruments used are: trocar and cannula, nasal speculum, uvula retractor and fiberoptic telescopes of differing angulation and a biopsy forceps [1, 6, 8] (fig. 5, 6).

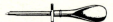

Trocar and Cannula for sinoscopy. Size: 5 mm.

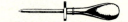

Trocar and Cannula for sinoscopy. Size: 4 mm.

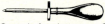

Trocar and Cannula for sinoscopy. Size: 3 mm.

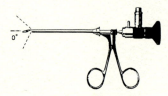

Biopsy Forceps with telescope

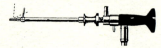

Uvula Retractor. For use with Examining Telescope.

Fig.5. Jazbi pediatric set for nasopharyngoscopy and sinoscopy (Karl Storz Endoscopy America, Inc., Los Angeles, and Karl Storz, Tuttlingen, West Germany).

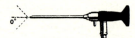

Straight Forward Examining Telescope.

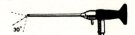

Forward-Oblique Examining Telescope.

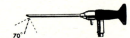

Lateral Examining Telescope.

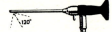

Retrospective Examining Telescope.

Attachment for Teaching
● Attaches to eyepiece of telescope.
● Simultaneous observation by operator and observer

Fig.6. Jazbi pediatric set for nasopharyngoscopy and sinoscopy (Karl Storz Endoscopy America, Inc., Los Angeles, and Karl Storz, Tuttlingen, West Germany).

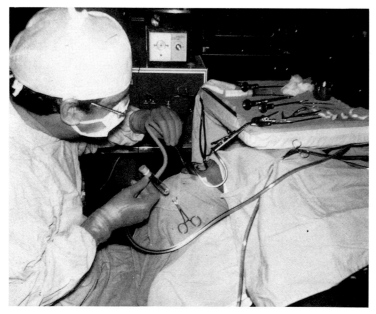

Fig.7. Collection of pus by pneumatic suction (see text for details).

Techniques

The technique is the same as used for antral puncture. Once the cavity of the sinus is reached the trocar is withdrawn and replaced by a fiberoptic telescope and the sinus cavity is examined under direct vision. The telescope can be moved up and down and at the same time can be rotated to obtain more accessability, allowing the entire cavity to be inspected by using telescopes of differing angulation [1, 3, 6, 8] (fig.6).

If pus or fluid is visualized it is aspirated either by a disposable 20-cm^3 syringe or by pneumatic suction whereby the pus is collected in a glass tube for culture and sensitivity [8] (fig.7). Culture of the aspirated purulent material is necessary to determine the precise organism as therapy is based upon this [8, 14]. The sinus cavity is examined again under direct vision by fiberoptic telescopes of varying degrees. 30 and 70° optics are useful for examining the sinus mucosa, however, a retrograde fiberoptic telescope of 120° is essential to visualize the maxillary ostium [1, 6, 8, 11]. In cases where a biopsy is desirable, it can be obtained under direct vision by using the biopsy forceps.

Nasopharyngoscopy

Nasopharyngoscopy is carried out with relative ease by using a specially designed retractor through which a fiberoptic telescope can be inserted and the nasopharynx examined under direct vision [8, 10] (fig. 5).

Teaching and Photography

For teaching purposes a specially designed 'teaching attachment' is used whereby an assistant or a resident can observe at the same time (fig. 6). If photographs are desirable, these can be obtained by using a robot camera or the new endo camera with a combined flash generator and light source. For instant color photos, polaroid camera is also available (available from Karl Storz Endoscopy, America, Inc. of Los Angeles, and Karl Storz of Tuttlingen, West Germany.)

In the beginning, it used to be rather cumbersome to take photographs but the new setup has not only eliminated the use of a cable, but has made it a lot easier and faster as the endo camera is considerably lighter than the robot camera and consequently much easier to handle (fig. 8, 9).

Repeated Irrigation

If repeated irrigations are deemed necessary the 'Jazbi maxillary sinus ventilation tube' (available from Xomed, Cincinnati, Ohio) is left in position which serves as an in-dwelling catheter (fig. 10). The ventilation tube is designed to stay in the maxillary sinus until it is pulled out by the physician. It has flexible wings at one end. These are bent and brought together manually for insertion through the cannula. Once the tube goes past the cannula

---

a–d: Nasopharyngoscopy

a: Showing adenoids. Posterior nares and post nasal drip.

b: Nasopharyngoscopy showing hypertrophied adenoids obstructing posterior nares. Note mucopus on adenoids and in the vicinity of eustachian tubes.

c: Showing adenoids, part of posterior nares, and opening of eustachian tube.

d: Showing choanae, openings of the eustachian tubes, and rhinopharynx after surgical removal of rhabdomyo sarcoma.

e–h: Sinoscopy

e: Sinoscopy before adenotonsillectomy. See text for details.

f: Mucopus in maxillary sinus (Chronic sinusitis).

g: Telescopic view of left maxillary sinus showing mucosal cyst near lateral wall roof of the maxillary sinus.

h: Telescopic view of right maxillary sinus showing opening of the natural ostium. Note a mucosal cyst along the floor of the sinus.

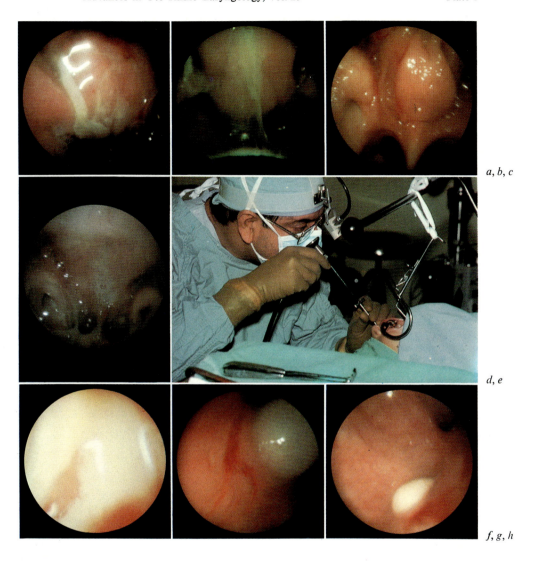

a, b, c

d, e

f, g, h

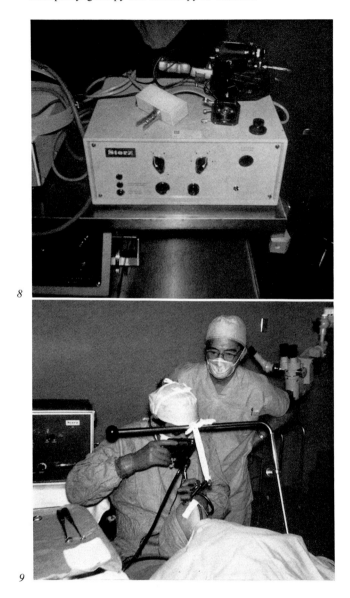

8

9

Fig.8. Robot camera and flash unit (Karl Storz Endoscopy America, Inc., Los Angeles, and Karl Storz, Tuttlingen, West Germany).

Fig.9. Endo camera and the new combined light source and flash (Karl Storz Endoscopy America, Inc., Los Angeles, and Karl Storz, Tuttlingen, West Germany).

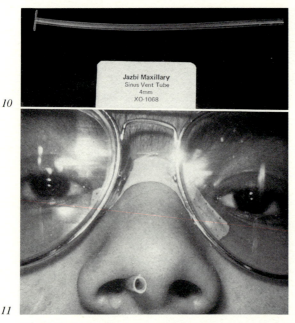

Jazbi Maxillary
Sinus Vent Tube
4mm
XO-1068

10

11

Fig. 10. Jazbi maxillary sinus ventilation tube (Xomed, Cincinnati, Ohio).
Fig. 11. Vent tube in position (pulled out for irrigation).

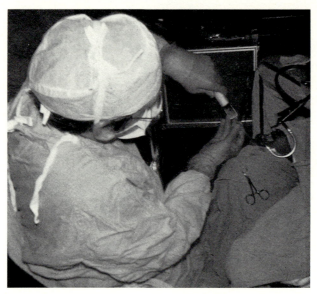

Fig. 12. Sinus irrigation by a disposable syringe via ventilation tube (see text).

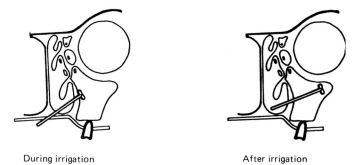

During irrigation   After irrigation

Fig.13. Position of the tube during and after irrigation.

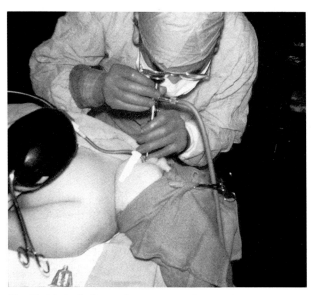

Fig.14. Method of nasopharyngoscopy (see text).

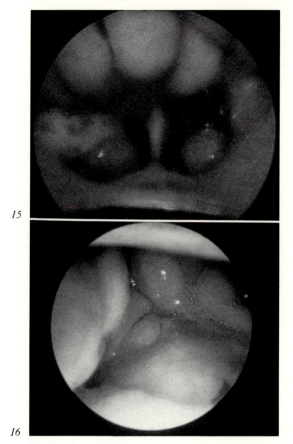

15

16

Fig. 15. A view through the nasopharyngoscope showing choanae and posterior ends of the inferior turbinates. Note mucopus on the left side.

Fig. 16. A view through the nasopharyngoscope showing adenoids and opening of the Eustachian tube.

and enters the sinus cavity, the wings flare open. At this time the cannula is also withdrawn leaving the tube in the maxillary sinus. The ventilation tube is gently pulled out until the wings hit the medial wall of the sinus cavity [8] (fig. 11).

Sinus irrigation is carried out by a syringe through the ventilation tube in the usual manner (fig. 12). Once this is done the tube is pushed back until it hits against the lateral wall of the sinus. The tube is cut at the level of the anterior nares and is tucked under the vestibule (fig. 13).

For subsequent irrigations the tube is pulled out by forceps until the wings hit the medial wall of the sinus. A number 12 or number 14 syringe needle or an adapter is introduced though the lumen of the tube depending upon the size of the tube, and irrigation carried out in the usual manner.

This method avoids repeated anesthesia and antral punctures. The tube can be pulled out by the physician with a pair of forceps without any difficulty. No anesthetic is necessary. If repeated irrigations fail to resolve infection, a Caldwell-Luc procedure merits consideration [8, 13, 16, 19].

Summary

Endoscopy of the maxillary sinus is very helpful not only in providing exact information regarding pathology in the antrum, but it also helps in the management of the condition by enabling us to make a correct diagnosis. The examination is easier and more reliable under direct vision rather than with an X-ray examination or antral puncture. The latest development and modification in the existing armamentarium have proved to be of great value in teaching because it not only allows to take color photographs but also affords an assistant or a student the opportunity to observe the procedure simultaneously through a teaching attachment. Likewise, in the nasopharynx, it is now easy to examine the entire nasopharynx for the presence of abnormal growth or some other pathology (fig. 14–16). It can be gainfully employed to check the pharyngeal end of the Eustachian tube for mechanical obstruction caused by adenoidal hypertrophy resulting in recurrent otitis media.

References

1   DRAF, W.: Wert der Sinoskopie für Klinik und Praxis. Z.Lar.Rhinol.Otol. *52:* 890–896 (1973).

2   GRAY, H.: Anatomy of the human body (Lea & Febiger, Philadelphia 1973).

3   GRUENBERG, H.: Die primär chronische Sinusitis maxillaris im endoskopischen Bild. Z.Lar.Rhinol.Otol. *50:* 813–817 (1971).

4   HELLMICH, S. und HERBERHOLDT, C.: Technische Verbesserungen der Kieferhöhlenendoskopie. Arch.Ohr.-Nas.-KehlkHeilk. *199:* 678–682 (1971).

5   HINDERER, K.H.: Nasal problems in children. Pediat.Ann. *5:* 499–509 (1975).

6   ILLUM. P. and JEPPESEN, F.: Sinoscopy: endoscopy of the maxillary sinus. Acta otolar. *73:* 506–512 (1972).

7 JAFFE, B.F.: Chronic sinusitis in children. Comments on pathogenesis and management. Clin. Pediat. *13:* 944–948 (1974).

8 JAZBI, B. and RITTER, F.N.: Sinoscopy and sinus disease in children. Otolar. Clins N. Am. *10:* 71–80 (1977).

9 MASING, H.: Surgery on the lateral nasal wall with the operation microscope. Rhinology *14:* 73–77 (1976).

10 MESSERKLINGER, W.: Nasenendoskopie. Der mittlere Nasengang und seine unspezifischen Entzündungen. HNO *20:* 212–215 (1972)

11 MESSERKLINGER, W.: Technik und Möglichkeiten der Nasenendoskopie. HNO *20:* 133–135 (1972).

12 PROCTOR, D.F. and ANDERSEN, I.: Nasal mucociliary function in normal man. Rhinology *14:* 11–17 (1976).

13 RAMON, Y.; OBERMAN, M.; FREEDMAN, A., and KALDERON, S.: The maxillary sinus. A surgical approach via a gingivomucoperiosteal flap. Archs Otolar. *102:* 637–639 (1976).

14 RITTER, F.: The paranasal sinuses. Anatomy and surgical technique (Mosby, St. Louis 1973).

15 SCHAEFFER, J.P.: The embryology, development and anatomy of the nose, paranasal sinuses, naso-lacrimal passageways and olfactory organ in man (Blakiston, Philadelphia 1920).

16 THOMSON, S.C. and NEGUS, V.E.: Maxillary sinusitis. Operation; Diseases of the nose and throat; 6th ed., chapter 16, pp. 244–249 (Cassell, London 1955).

17 VAN ALYEA, O.E.: Nasal sinuses. An anatomic and clinical consideration (Williams & Wilkins, Baltimore 1951).

18 WILSON, T.G.: Acute rhinitis and sinusitis; in Diseases of the ear, nose and throat in children (Heinemann, London 1962).

19 RITTER, F.N.: A clinical and anatomical study of the various techniques of irrigation of the maxillary sinus. Laryngoscope *87:* 215–223 (1977).

20 SIMPSON, J.F.; ROBIN, I.C.; BALLANTYNE, J.C., and GROVES, J.: A synopsis of otolaryngology (Wright, Bristol 1967).

B. JAZBI, MD, DLO, FAAP, Professor and Chief of Otorhinolaryngology, University of Missouri, Kansas City, School of Medicine, The Children's Mercy Hospital, *Kansas City, MO 64108* (USA)

Adv. Oto-Rhino-Laryng., vol. 23, pp. 87–96 (Karger, Basel 1978)

Examination of the Pediatric Upper Airway with the Flexible Nasopharyngolaryngoscope

HARVEY D. SILBERMAN and JOHN A. TUCKER

Background

The examination of the pediatric larynx and nasopharynx, any place other than an operating room, can be a stressful if not an impossible procedure.

In 1970, we added the flexible fibreoptic bronchoscope to our endoscopic inventory. As our technique mainly utilized transnasal introduction, it became evident that the flexible bronchoscope afforded an examination of the nasopharynx and larynx with little discomfort or stimulation of the gag reflex. This led to the occasional use in the office of the flexible bronchoscope for nasopharyngoscopy and laryngoscopy. It was particularly reassuring to be able to view the larynx in those patients whose laryngeal mirror examination was inadequate. Others have had a similar experience [1, 2]. Thus, it was unnecessary to expose the patient's larynx a rigid laryngoscope in a hospital setting. The same was true for those patients in whom the nasopharynx was not adequately accessible to the small nasopharyngeal mirror or the nasopharyngoscope.

The flexible bronchoscope not only allowed an excellent view, but at the same time was more comfortable than the standard methods. Simple topical anesthesia was quite sufficient for a more than adequate examination of the nasopharynx and larynx.

The main drawback of using this instrument in the pediatric patient was of course the large diameter. The use of the flexible bronchoscope in the large child was really no problem, but it was out of the question in the smaller child. The Olympus Optical Company has had available for several years a pediatric flexible bronchoscope which had the ideal outer diameter, but was much too long (60 vm, effective length, with a total length of 77 cm) and certainly rather expensive for office use. Its diameter is an ideal 3.7 mm. It has 68° of forward viewing. The depth of field is 3 mm to infinity. Unfortunately, the cost and length, which made it much too cumbersome for office procedures, precluded its use. Of note was a tip deflection of 180° upwards and 30° downwards.

Approximately 3 years ago, a flexible fibreoptic laryngoscope, introduced by the American Optical Company, designed for anesthesia intubation, became commercially available [3]. The instrument was quite inexpensive. It was 49 cm long (effective length, not including controls) and 6.25 mm in diameter. It had a controllable tip with a total deflection of 120°. The field of view was 60° and the depth of focus 5–30 mm. The total length of the instrument was 67 cm.

Immediately upon receipt of this instrument it became apparent that it could not be used in children because of its large diameter. In addition it had poor optics and was quite clumsy with which to work. This scope, however, was adequate for its intended purpose, that being intubation in the adult.

Another flexible laryngoscope had also been designed in 1972 for anesthesia needs but again was too wide for otolaryngology's use [4].

It was apparent that a need existed for a scope primarily designed for otolaryngology. With the aid of the Machida Endoscope Company (Machida America, Inc.) such an instrument was produced to our specifications and desires.

A prototype instrument underwent clinical trial in May of 1975. Between May and December of that year, the prototype had been used in over 1,000 pediatric and adult patients in both the office and hospital setting.

The prototype scope weighed 6 oz. and was 20 cm long (effective length). The diameter was 3.9 mm. The diameter must be kept below 4 mm to allow passage through the nasal cavity from newborn through adulthood (fig. 1).

The diameter of 3.9 mm limits the flexibility of the tip to 90° in the downward direction, but that is quite sufficient. This lightweight, highly flexible and relatively short scope allows for 360° rotation in any direction without patient discomfort.

With a scope of these dimensions, we finally had an instrument that could be of use in the pediatric patient. Biopsy of the larynx with this scope in children was not even a consideration. Certainly biopsy of the larynx through a flexible instrument is difficult, undependable. In the child without an adequate airway could prove fatal.

There is an obvious absence of a biopsy-aspirating channel in our flexible scope. The reason for this is twofold.

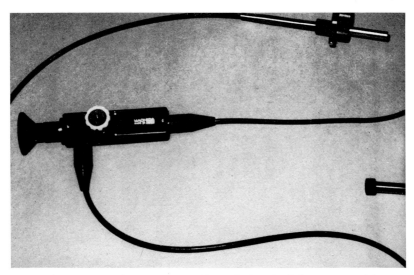

Fig. 1. The prototype instrument was 20 cm in length. Subsequent models were 25 cm in length and 3.9 mm in diameter.

First, at this stage in the state of the art of flexible instruments, as previously mentioned, biopsy should not be done.

Secondly, there is normally great ease in anesthetizing topically the nasopharyngeal-laryngeal area. The older child has the ability to clear mucous in the nose and throat by merely sniffing, blowing his nose and swallowing. In the infant, there is almost an instinctive swallowing which occurs with the introduction of the scope.

The prototype length was 20 cm. Subsequent models were increased to 25 cm. Consideration to make it longer was dropped as we definitely did not desire to recreate a preexisting instrument (Olympus), which did not fill our specifications.

Weight has been held to a minimum 6 oz. This allows extreme ease of handling and manipulation. The control knob is so situated to permit tip angulation, by simply moving one's thumb.

Despite the decrease in diameter of the scope, the optical bundle has been doubled in size in comparison to the standard Machida flexible bronchoscope. The image is therefore superior to the large Machida bronchoscope. When compared to rigid nasopharyngoscopes and laryngoscopes designed for similar purposes, the flexible nasopharyngolaryngoscope fairs quite well, especially with a field of vision of 70° and a depth of focus of 5–50 mm.

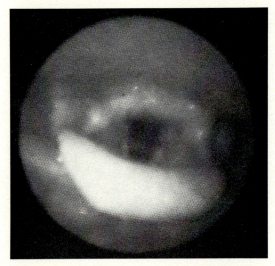

Fig. 2. The larynx is in a 'natural' state not artificially suspendend by the blade of an anterior commissure laryngoscope.

Clinical Application

The nasopharyngolaryngoscope was designed not as a replacement for our routine methods of examining the nasopharynx and larynx, but as an adjunct. This instrument allows one to examine completely all patients, including those in whom the routine methods are not adequate. It has been found that the 3.9-mm diameter will fit most full-term newborn nasal chambers. The flexible scope allows us to rule out choanal atresia and at the same time perform nasopharyngoscopy and laryngoscopy.

Examination of the pediatric larynx with this instrument allows a rather unique experience. The larynx is in a 'natural' state, not artificially suspended by the blade of a laryngoscope (fig. 2).

Flexible examination of newborns with stridorous respirations has been found to be unusually easy. One can easily observe the floppy epiglottis or other pathologic lesions of the larynx which may exist.

Of late, we have been using the flexible scope in the diagnosis of acute epiglottitis. This of course is always a controversial subject. However, the use of this instrument has been an enormous help. Again, its use has been adjunctive. We pass the scope in the usual transnasal mode. This avoids stimulation of the gag reflex or coughing which is paramount in the management of acute epiglottitis.

With the scope suspended at about the level of the soft palate, we are able to view the epiglottis with relative impunity, and make our diagnosis.

It must be stressed at this point that this is a new modality and despite our expertise with it, we have a laryngoscope and open tube bronchoscope at our side.

Routine daily examination of the epiglottis is carried out with the flexible nasopharyngolaryngoscope so that we might determine the optimum time for extubation of children with acute epiglottitis.

Another extremely valuable aspect of this intrument is its use in nasopharyngeal and laryngeal examination of school age children. It is well recognized there is a great difficulty in examining the nasopharynx and larynx in this age group. No longer do we have to depend upon X-ray, digital examination, or examination under general anesthesia to evaluate the nasopharynx.

We are able to employ this technique to also aid in ruling out the presence or absence of velopharyngeal incompetence.

Despite the fact the use of this instrument has become routine in our pediatric pratice, we do not in any way suggest that it can be used in every child in the office setting. The age group from 3 to 6 years may prove difficult if not impossible and will require an operating room examination. We have found that in the operating room away from the parents, the flexible scope can be used without general anesthesia.

Technique of Introduction of the Flexible Nasopharyngolaryngoscope

In children requiring examination of the nasopharynx and larynx, the scope is routinely passed transnasally. It is by far the most comfortable method for the patient and permits complete examination of the entire upper airway with one introduction (fig. 3).

The nose is anesthetized topically. The topical chosen is not that important except that it be rapid and employ an epinephrine-like drug to cause shrinkage of the nasal mucosa. We introduce applicator sticks dipped in the anesthetic. The applicators are placed on the floor of the nose and progressively advanced towards the nasopharynx. Usually the oropharynx is sprayed topically. There is often so little stimulation of the gag reflex that even this step can be omitted.

The scope is slid along the floor of the nose after the applicators are removed. Examination of the nasal chambers is geatly facilitated with the

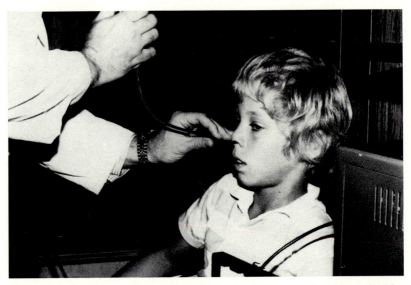

Fig. 3. The scope is passed transnasally. It is by far the most comfortable method for the patient.

nasopharyngolaryngoscope. One is able to inspect beneath each turbinate and high into the spheno-ethmoidal recess in the larger child. Visualization of the sphenoid ostia is also readily accomplished in those noses large enough.

The nasopharynx and Eustachian orifice comes shortly into view. Upon reaching the posterior septum, the scope is turned on its side and the tip angled to allow one to visualize the contralateral Eustachian tube orifice. Virtually all anatomical areas of the nasopharynx including the fossa of Rosenmuller are well visualized.

Biopsy of the nasopharynx in the older child is a reality accomplished with a degree of comfort and accuracy not previously possible. Unlike the larynx, this area is fixed and does not freely move. The technique consists of passing the scope, unter topical anesthesia, locating the lesion and then passing the biopsy forceps through the ipsalateral or contralateral nares. The lesion is then biopsied under direct visualization. If bleeding should ensue, this area can be easily cauterized electrically or chemically under direct observation.

After examination of the nose and nasopharynx, the patient is instructed to breathe through his nose. This allows the soft palate to fall away from the posterior nasopharyngeal wall. This is an excellent time to observe velo-pharyngeal closure. To accomplish this, simply have the child phonate. With

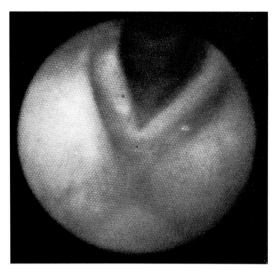

Fig.4. We are able to view the anterior commissure with a facility not previously possible in the office setting.

the palate relaxed, one is able to examine the posterior aspect of the soft palate and uvula.

Almost immediately, the base of the tongue, vallecula, epiglottis, and larynx come into view. The scope is advanced to the level of the oropharynx, just above the epiglottis. One is immediately impressed by the lack of stimulation of the gag reflex by this route of introduction.

The shape of the epiglottis and the presence of anatomical abnormalities are in no way a problem. Thus far, no larynx has been examined in which the entire laryngeal area could not be seen. Certainly, this cannot be said of the laryngeal mirror in the child. Any mucous that may accumulate on the tip of the instrument can be simply cleared by having the child swallow, using the epiglottis 'as a windshield wiper'.

Once the larynx is in view, it is possible to see the laryngeal surface of the epiglottis and anterior commissure. Without discomfort to the patient, one is able to observe the larynx for an extended length of time, watching him swallow and cough without need to remove the scope. Observation of this degree was not previously available in the office (fig.4).

As we alluded to before, there are some children in whom it is impossible to pass the flexible nasopharyngolaryngoscope in the office. These children must be done in the operating room. The examination differs, however, from the routine laryngeal examination using an anterior commissure laryngoscope. The anesthesia varies from simple light sedation to insufflation without intubation. The type of course depends upon the child and your individual department of anesthesia. With the child under anesthesia, an extremely complete examination of the nasopharynx and larynx can be carried out with the flexible scope. The field of view is enormous compared to the relative tunnel vision that we have with the standard pediatric anterior commissure scope.

It becomes apparent that at 25 cm in length, the nasopharyngolaryngo-scope could easily be used as a bronchoscope in the smaller child. We would take this opportunity to warn those not totally familiar with management and examination of pediatric airways that this could lead to serious compli-cations. This is due to the relative size of the pediatric airway, and the degree of obstruction offered by a truly solid flexible scope.

Special Uses of the Flexible Nasopharyngolaryngoscope

Newborn nursery. It is quite conceivable that the flexible nasopharyngo-laryngoscope someday will become a standard part of every newborn physi-cal examination. One can immediately discern if a choanal atresia is present and if the nasopharynx and larynx are normal. This of course brings about another problem, that being, who should perform the examination – the laryngologist or the pediatrician? Obviously, it is our strong belief that the pediatrician should not employ this instrument. Our reason being that like all things with great potential good there is great potential danger. The laryngologist is eminently more qualified to handle airway problems than is the pediatrician. In the hands of those inadequately trained, airway tragedies will undoubtedly occur, and disease entities will be missed.

Bedside laryngoscopy and nasopharyngoscopy. Examination of the bed-ridden child has often been a problem. Cooperation in an extremely ill child as we all know is frequently impossible. With this new scope, the examina-tion is readily accomplished. One merely requires the scope, a light source and a small amount of topical anesthesia. Full cooperation of the child is only secondary (fig. 5).

Inability to open the mouth. Not infrequently one is faced with the child who cannot despite cooperative attempts, open his mouth. Such would

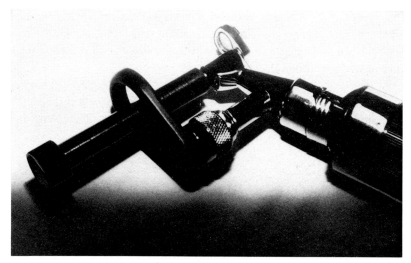

Fig.5. One may use an adapter for a halogen light otoscope which will aid in emergency use of the flexible nasopharyngolaryngoscope.

be a child who has sustained multiple facial fractures and has required wiring of the mandible. If a laryngeal problem were to appear in such a child, examination of the larynx could at least be performed without removing the wires.

Photography. Photographic documentation is invaluable. The system employed with the flexible nasopharyngolaryngoscope is rather unique. It requires two additional pieces of equipment besides the scope. They are the camera and the light source.

Our camera is a specially constructed single lens reflex, the Kowa SQ16 (Machida America, Inc.), using the 110 instamatic format. The light source ist the Machida xenon light, model RN-300F, with built-in strobe. One merely pulls the shutter release on the motor-driven camera for excellent pictures. The automation is entirely built into the camera and light source.

Despite the small format, the resulting pictures are quite adequate and probably are as good or better than the best existing systems.

At the present time, we have also been using a 35-mm format. This consists of a Pentax single lens reflex camera with a 135-mm telephoto lens and a Machida adapter. We have been using high speed Ektachrome film and the Machida xenon light source. For the moment, the Kowa camera is preferred because of its much smaller size.

Teaching aid. There is available a teaching sidearm which can be placed on the nasopharyngolaryngoscope. The sidearm is an invaluable teaching aid. One can in a step by step manner teach students and residents the living anatomy of the upper airway.

Sinoscopy. In those children who for one reason or another have had their sinuses opened surgically, follow-up examination of the sinus interior can be performed as an outpatient.

Positioning and patency of endotracheal and tracheotomy tubes. The flexible scope can be passed through most endotracheal tubes and tracheotomy tubes. We are more and more frequently doing routine examinations of the tracheotomy tube and the trachea following tracheotomy to insure an adequate airway.

Passage through endotracheal tubes, 4.5 mm inside diameter and larger, can easily be carried out. This facilitates quick checks for position of the tubes and is virtually routine in our hospital.

Comment

A new practical instrument and technique for examing the pediatric airway has been introduced. It allows for a completeness of examination not previously possible in all cases as an office or bedside procedure. The ease of examination and patient tolerance make for a remarkable new clinical experience.

References

1   DAVIDSON, T.M.; BONE, R.C., and NAHUM, A.M.: Flexible fiberoptic laryngo-bronchoscopy. Laryngoscope, *84:* 1876–1882 (1974).
2   DELLON, A.L.; HALL, C.A., and CHRETIEN, P.B.: Fibreoptic endoscopy in the head and neck region. Plastic reconstr. Surg. *55:* 466–71 (1975).
3   DAVIS, N.J.: A new fiberoptic laryngoscope for nasal intubation. Anesth. Analg. J., *52* (1973).
4   STILES, C.M.; STILES, R., and DENSON, J.S.: A flexible fibreoptic laryngoscope. J. Am. med. Ass. *221* (1972).

H.D. SILBERMAN, MD, Clinical Assistant Professor of Otorhinology, Temple University, School of Medicine, 6905 Castor Ave., *Philadelphia, PA 19149* (USA)

Adv. Oto-Rhino-Laryng., vol. 23, pp. 97–103 (Karger, Basel 1978)

Management of Subglottic Stenosis of the Larynx in Infants and Children

BLAIR FEARON

Department of Otolaryngology, Hospital for Sick Children, and The University of Toronto Faculty of Medicine, Toronto

The laryngeal subglottis, as described by BRYCE [1] is a space bounded below by the inferior margin of the cricoid cartilage and above by the insertion of the fibres of the elastic lamina into the vocal cords. Subglottic stenosis may be defined as a circumferential narrowing of this space, either by fibrous tissue alone, or by an abnormally small or underdeveloped cricoid ring, or because the cricoid cartilage is abnormally thick.

The definition of subglottic stenosis presents a problem. In 1932, TUCKER [2] stated that the cricoid lumen of a normal newborn infant is 6 mm in diameter. In 1972, FEARON and COTTON [3] reported that the normal effective lumen of the subglottic space to be 4.5 mm. The extent of the stenosis may vary from a thin fibrous web-like membrane to involvement of the total subglottic space. Furthermore, in either acquired or congenital stenosis, the subglottic space and one or more of the tracheal rings may be incorporated in the lesion.

Subglottic Stenosis

Congenital

HOLINGER et al. [4] reported that in 158 patients with subglottic stenosis, 115 were congenital and 43 were acquired. In our own series of 35 patients, 29 appeared to be congenital in origin [5]. In a newborn intensive care unit, PARKIN et al. [6] reported 18 out of 603 admissions as subglottic stenosis, 3 of which were considered to be congenital and the remainder acquired.

Acquired

Acquired subglottic stenosis is caused by trauma, either internal, e.g. inhalation of heat or caustics, endotracheal tubes, or external trauma, e.g. sharp or blunt injuries such as HIGH tracheotomy. As far back as 1916, TURNER [7] reported stenoses of the larynx in children following intubation. Since a report by MACDONALD and STOCKS [8] in 1965, in which prolonged nasal intratracheal intubation was advocated for the management of airway insufficiency, the problem of subglottic stenosis as well as other laryngeal pathology [9] have become much more prevalent. The author has seen total obliteration of the subglottic space after only 36 h of intubation [10]. Recently, HOLINGER *et al.* [4] and PARKIN *et al.* [6] have discussed in considerable detail the factors in the production of acquired subglottic stenosis.

Diagnosis of Congenital Subglottic Stenosis

Congenital subglottic stenosis is not always apparent at birth, although when it is, stridor is the most common symptom. This is a to-and-fro sound, but when the stenosis is severe, it is accompanied by dyspnoea and a croupy cough. Cyanosis may develop, especially when the child is crying. On the other hand, symptoms may not develop until the child has a respiratory infection and then the picture is very similar to that of an acute laryngotracheitis. In fact, some patients are treated repeatedly for croup before the correct diagnosis is realized. Occasionally, the diagnosis is only apparent when an attempt is made to pass an endotracheal tube for the purpose of giving a general anaesthetic for some surgical procedure.

Although xerography and tomography are useful adjuncts to the diagnosis of subglottic stenosis, at times these may be misleading. Direct laryngoscopy and bronchoscopy are essential for the accurate assessment of the degree and of the extent of the stenosis. The critical decision is whether or not to pass a bronchoscope through a stenosis that may be adequate for respiratory exchange when the child is healthy, although the same size opening may not be adequate should the child have a respiratory infection. Our philosophy is that if passing a suitably sized bronchoscope [11], e.g. a 3-mm bronchoscope in a newborn child is likely to precipitate a tracheotomy, then the child's life would be in jeopardy anyway. On the other hand, a stenosis may be thin enough to dilate with bronchoscopes and the airway thereby improved to the degree that the child's respiratory exchange is normal. In 8 of 29 patients with congenital subglottic stenosis, we were able

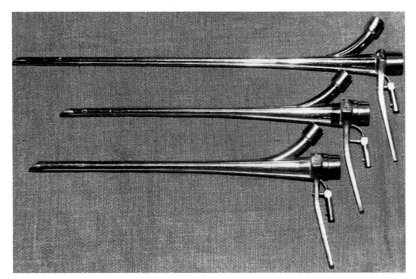

Fig. 1. Two special scopes and a standard 3 × 26 Holinger bronchoscope.

to dilate the stenosis successfully with one or more procedure so that not only was the tracheotomy unnecessary, but the patients no longer had signs of stenosis [5].

The initial management of congenital subglottic stenosis is determined by the functional lumen of the subglottic space, the length of the stenosis, and whether or not there are other concomitant abnormalities in the patient. The first consideration is whether a tracheotomy is necessary to sustain adequate ventilation of the patient – not only when the health of the child is good, but also whether the airway will be adequate if the child has a respiratory infection.

Diagnosis of Acquired Subglottic Stenosis

The length of time in which an endotracheal tube may be left in place without causing damage to the larynx is controversial, but there is still no hard and fast method of determining how long an endotracheal tube may be in place without developing a stenosis. Neither is there any means of determining in advance whether or not a severe stenosis will respond to dilatations. By experience, we have found that if dilatations are instituted before the fibrous stage has developed, even if there is a total closure of the sub-glottic space, an adequate lumen can be achieved by repeated dilatations [12]. As with any fibrous stenosis, dilatations must be carried out properly or else no improvement, even a worsening of the problem may result. The goal is to stretch the fibrous tissue without causing any undue trauma. We prefer to carry out serial dilatations with graduated sizes of bronchoscopes [11]. The Pilling Company of Philadelphia has made for us a special type of subglottic-tracheoscopes, designed for the purpose of both examining the subglottic space and the trachea, as well as for a dilatation. These are really modifications of the Holinger or Jackson bronchoscopes (fig. 1). These are 3-, 3.5-, 4-, and 5-mm bronchoscopes shortened to a length of 20 cm and made without fenestres. To use these for dilation, the tip is directed into the stenosis and advanced in a spiral movement of the instrument. This achieves a maximum dilating effect with the least trauma, although if the lumen of the stenosis is very small, as an adjunct to the dilatation with the scopes, Jackson laryngeal dilators are used.

Surgical Correction of Subglottic Stenosis

At best, the child with a severe subglottic stenosis is committed to long periods of hospitalization in his formative years, enduring repeated dila-tations and creating a tremendous financial burden on the family and to the community. These patients live a hazardous existence, for in spite of most meticulous nursing care and medical attention, death can occur rapidly and unexpectedly [3].

In 1971, GRAHNE [11] in Finland reported an operative procedure to correct severe chronic traumatic laryngeal stenosis in 7 cases under 3 years of age. This operation involved a laryngofissure type of approach in which a median section of the thyroid and cricoid cartilages as well as the upper most tracheal rings is performed. The ring of cicatricial stenosis is resected completely. This is followed by a median section of the mucosa and the posterior cricoid lamina down to the esophageal musculature with or without sectioning the interarytenoid muscles. An Aboulker prothesis of a suitable size is introduced so that it extends from above the vocal cords to below the tracheotomy level in the trachea. The prothesis is maintained in position for 4 months by wiring a tracheotomy tube through a hole in the prothesis. The posterior incision in the lamina is not closed, but the larynx and anterior wall of the trachea are closed with catgut and silk. The results in the 7 cases were reported as being excellent. However, one would wonder whether such an extensive procedure was justified in all of these patients in view of the fact that 2 of them had not required a tracheotomy at all, and one only temporarily before the Grahne operation was performed. We believe the operation has a great deal of merit, but should be reserved for those patients in whom a less extensive procedure as the one described below, has failed.

For more than a period of 20 years, the author has tried unsuccessfully to correct subglottic stenosis by various means of internal stenting. Finally, a successful result was achieved by transecting anteriorly the cricoid cartilage with its underlying fibrous stenosis and placing an interpositional graft or rib cartilage between the cut ends of the cricoid [10]. Although we found this rib graft difficult to maintain in position, nonetheless, the lumen was improved sufficiently that the patient could be extubated.

The Fearon-Cotton Operation for Correction of Subglottic Stenosis

While listening to a paper by LAPIDOT et al. [12] on the use of thyroid cartilage to replace the cricoid cartilage in piglets, it occurred to us that a portion of the thyroid cartilage could be used as an interpositional graft between the cut ends of the divided cricoid. By leaving this graft partially attached to its origin, we theorized that the graft would be easier to retain in position. With the financial assistance from the Medical Research Council of Canada and with the assistance of Dr. R. COTTON, as a research fellow, a feasibility study was undertaken, using growing monkeys (African Green) as a research model to determine: (1) whether removing a piece of cartilage from the thyroid ala and whether dividing the cricoid cartilage anteriorly would interfere with the function and development of the larynx; (2) if such a flap could be rotated into position between the cut ends of the cricoid, and (3) if the graft would 'take' and thus enlarge the cricoid lumen. It was shown that in these experiments the growth and function of the larynx were not impaired; that a rotation flap could be used successfully; and that the lumen of the cricoid was enlarged satisfactorily. An unexpected finding was that the monkeys in which a simple anterior section of the cricoid allowed the latter to develop into the form of a 'U' as it grew, thus enlarging the lumen without an anterior interpositional graft [3], [9]. Because the results on this experimental surgery were more than satisfactory, it was decided to employ the same method on patients with severe subglottic stenoses that were failing to respond to dilatation.

Under general anaesthesia via the pre-existing tracheotomy, the laryn-geal and upper tracheal cartilages are exposed by a collar incision centred on the cricoid cartilage. The anterior lamina of the cricoid is split in or near the midline and this incision may be extended downwards to include the upper tracheal rings, depending on the extent of the stenosis. No attempt is made to reduce the bulk of the fibrous tissue present within the lumen of the cricoid and no internal stenting or surfacing is used. In spite of the feasibility of rotating a thyroid cartilaganeous flap in the animal experiments, it has not been possible because of extensive fibrosis, to leave the thyrochondral flap attached to the thyroid cartilage. In other words, a free graft taken from the lower third of the thyroid cartilage has been used. In patients neither with extensive tracheal stenosis, it may not be feasible to use the thyro-chondral graft, but one may have to resort to using a piece of rib cartilage. The graft is placed between the cut ends of the cricoid lamina and the in-volved tracheal rings and fixed in position with 5–0 Prolene sutures. The soft tissues are then approximated in the midline, a Penrose string inserted and the skin closed with either a subcuticular wire or heavy subcuticular Der-malon suture.

An annoying problem that has delayed the decannulation in some pa-tients is that of a flap of the anterior tracheal wall protruding into the tracheal lumen, because of the cephalad traction of the tracheotomy tube in patients with short necks. This can be overcome by using a second tape attached to the plate of the trachotomy tube, passed under the arms and tied at the back of the patient [10].

Five of the first 7 patients in which the Fearon-Cotton technique has been used have been decannulated. The extent of the stenosis in the other 2 was really far too great to expect this procedure to be successful and, in fact, each of the latter 2 have had additional surgery in which a variation of the Grahne technique has been used. The operation in both of these children has been too recent to determine the end result. Another 2 patients have had the Fearon-Cotton procedure carried out, but they also are too early to be evaluated.

A new modality of treatment has been instituted recently in which the carbon dioxide gas laser has been used to divide a subglottic stenosis, as well as a tracheal stenosis. As yet, our experience has been too limited, but nevertheless we believe that the laser has great potential in treating patients with certain types of webs or with troublesome complications, such as granulomata [5].

References

1   BRYCE, D.P.: The laryngeal subglottis. J.Lar.Otol. *89:* 667 (1975).

2   TUCKER, G.: The infant larynx; direct laryngoscopic observations. J.Am.med.Ass. *99:* 1899 (1932).

3   FEARON, B. and COTTON, R.: Subglottic stenosis in infants and children; the clinical problem and the experimental surgical correction. Can.J.Otolaryng. *1:* 281 (1972).

4   HOLINGER, P.; SCHILD, J.; KUTNICK, S., and HOLINGER, L.: Subglottic stenosis in infants and children. Ann.Otol.Rhinol.Lar.*85:* 591 (1976).

5   FEARON, B. and CINNAMOMD, M.: Surgical correction of subglottic stenosis of the larynx; clinical results of the Fearon-Cotton operation. Ann.Otol.Rhinol.Otol.*5:* 475 (1976).

6   PARKIN, J.L.; STEVENS, M.H., and JUNG, A.: Acquired and congenital subglottic stenosis in the infant. Ann.Otol.Rhinol.Lar.*85:* 573 (1976).

7   TURNER, A.L.: Stenosis of the larynx in children following intubation and tracheotomy. J.Otol.Laryng.*31:* 313 (1916).

8   McDONALD, I. and STOCKS, J.: Prolonged nasotracheal intubation. Br.J.Anaesth. *37:* 161 (1965).

9   FEARON, B. and COTTON, R.: Surgical correction of subglottic stenosis of the larynx. Preliminary report of an experimental surgical technique. Ann.Otol.Rhinol.Lar. *81:* 508 (1972).

10 FEARON, B. and ELLIS, D.: The management of long-term airway problems in infants and children. Ann.Otol.Rhinol.Lar.*80:* 669 (1971).

11 GRAHNE, B.: Operative treatment of severe chronic traumatic laryngeal stenosis in infants up to three years. Acta oto-lar.*72:* 134 (1971).

12 LAPIDOT, A.; SODAGAR, R., and RATANAPRASHTPORN, S.: Experimental repair of subglottic stenosis in piglets. Archs Otolar.*88:* 529 (1968).

13 FEARON, B. and COTTON, R.: Surgical correction of subglottic stenosis of the larynx in children. Progress report. Ann.Otol.Rhinol.Lar. *83:* 428 (1974).

B. FEARON, BA, MD, FRCS (C), FACS, Department of Otolaryngology, Hospital for Sick Children, *Toronto* (Canada)

Adv. Oto-Rhino-Laryng., vol. 23, pp. 104–108 (Karger, Basel 1978)

Lye Burns of the Esophagus and their Treatments

Frank N. Ritter

Department of Otorhinolaryngology, University of Michigan Center and
St. Joseph Mercy Hospital, Ann Arbor, Mich.

Introduction

Most caustics which are ingested are alkali. Acids are sometimes ingested and usually burn the stomach and pyloric region, so rarely come to attention of the otolaryngologist. Alkali damage to the oral cavity and the esophagus is not uncommon and has been managed by the otolaryngologist in the past.

The management of a patient who has ingested a caustic has never been by a precise group of guidelines because the amount and type of caustic swallowed, its concentration, and whether the patient had eaten before the ingestion are variables that, in general, produce different degrees of burns. Thus, each ingestion is accessed and managed individually.

The Effective of Alkali upon Tissues

Alkali damages tissue in the same way that heat causes a thermal burn. In burns of the food passages, a first degree burn is characterized by superficial loss of mucosa. A second degree burn involves the deeper tissues with damage to all layers. In a third degree burn, penetration beyond the organ occurs and peripheral tissues are also involved. As regards the oral cavity and esophagus, first degree burns are usually not serious, but second and third degree burns can result in strictures and even death.

Chemically, alkali causes fats and proteins to saponify and blood vessels to thrombose. This chemical reaction fixes the alkali to the tissues which thwarts any attempt to neutralize it by surface irrigation. Thus, deep penetration occurs and full thickness damage commonly results.

Solid Alkali Burns

Initially, after a patient ingests a solid caustic, usually swallowed in pellet form, the punctate burning which occurs, causes such pain that the patient does not often swallow additional caustic. Expectoration becomes a spontaneous symptom of ingestion, if the ingestion was done in an accidental manner. Fortunately, this protective action often prevents the patient from sustaining further damage. Then, the patient usually tries to drink water in an effort to modify the burning, which tends to neutralize any remaining caustic and washes it into the stomach, if it is not fixed to the tissues, where it can be neutralized by the gastric acids.

Diagnosis

The patient who ingests the solid caustic will first sustain burns of the anterior part of the oral cavity, and depending upon the amount swallowed, the pharynx and esophagus. Within 24 h, a leukocytic membrane can be noted at the point of each burn. A lipoidal study of the esophagus should be done to rule perforation and esophagoscopy should be diagnostically performed to see how severely the pharynx, larynx, and esophagus are damaged. It is advisable to wait at least 15 h after the burn has occurred in order for the leukocytic membrane to develop, as this makes easier identification of the burn by noting the leukocytic membrane. After 48 h, the risk of perforation is such that esophagoscopy is hazardous, so it is then best to assume that an esophageal burn has occurred and treat the patient without performing an esophagoscopy.

During esophagoscopy, the esophagus is instrumented until the first burn is encountered. Once that is noted, the esophagoscopy is terminated to prevent perforation. However, there is merit to doing a complete esophagoscopy, if it can be done safely because this provides a knowledge of the full extent of the burned area. Any remaining caustic can also be removed by lavage. Usually, a nasogastric tube is inserted for alimentation at esophagoscopy.

Treatment

Since 1964, steroids and antibiotics have been employed successfully in combination to reduce scar and stricture formation. In children, usually, 1 mg/kg of prednisone is used for 14 days, and then tapered over an 8-day period. Penicillin, in adequate dosage form to prevent infection, should also be continued during this 3 weeks. After 3 weeks, esophagoscopy is done.

materials to be marketed in a less concentrated amount and requiring the containers to be constructed in such a way to make them childproof. Further, education of the public on the corrosive nature of these materials has warned them of the extensive damage likely to be sustained if they are ingested. Initially, a great deal of experience was gained with solid caustic ingestion and the effects from it being isolated structure formation. Esophagoscopy, steroids and antibiotics, and repeated dilatations of the antegrade type, have been effective in minimizing damage of the esophagus.

Liquid alkali, which was initially marketed in the mid-1960s, caused severe damage to the entire upper gastrointestinal tract, from the lips to the pylorus. The Hazardous Substance Art has required modification of alkalin material and at the present time, has resulted in a weaker solution. While initially, esophagogastrectomy was an advocated treatment, perhaps, antibiotics and dilatations are now preferential treatment, unless severe strictures occur when esophagectomy is recommended.

References

1   ASHCRAFT, K.W. and PADULA, R.: The effect of dilute corrosives on the esophagus. Pediatrics *53:* 226 (1974).
2   RITTER, F.; NEWMAN, M.H., and NEWMAN, D.E.: A clinical and experimental study of corrosive burns of the stomach. Ann. Otol. Rhinol. Lar. *77:* 830 (1968).
3   KIRSH, M.M. and RITTER, F.N.: Caustic ingestion and subsequent damage to the oropharyngeal and digestive passages. Ann. thorc. Surg. *21:* 74 (1976).

F.N. RITTER, MD, Clinical Professor, Department of Otorhinolaryngology, University of Michigan Center and St. Joseph Mercy Hospital, *Ann Arbor, MI 48103* (USA)

Adv. Oto-Rhino-Laryng., vol. 23, pp. 109–114 (Karger, Basel 1978)

Suction Tonsillectomy

A Simplified Technique

Basharat Jazbi and Stephen Liston

Department of Otorhinolaryngology, University of Missouri, Kansas City, School of Medicine, Kansas City, Mo.

It is estimated that about 1,000,000 tonsillectomies and adenoidectomies are performed each year in the United States. Even though it is such a common procedure, there is considerable controversy about the indications for tonsillectomy and about the benefits gained from the operation. At present there is insufficient scientific information to answer many of the important questions about tonsillectomy. Some of these answers may be forthcoming from the result which will be obtained by the Workshop on Tonsillectomy and Adenoidectomy [1]. The procedure is not without its complications. The mortality of tonsillectomy and adenoidectomy is about 1 in 16,000 procedures [2]. Much of the mortality and morbidity of the operation is associated with bleeding. Despite the controversy there is no doubt that when properly performed, for adequate indications tonsillectomy can be of great benefit to the patient [3].

We believe that when the operation is performed, it should be done under optimal conditions. The use of this suction dissector makes the procedure safer and more controlled because intraoperative bleeding does not obscure the surgical landmarks. The instrument is extremely useful when teaching the technic of the operation. The bleeding is particularly unnerving to the neophyte surgeon and makes the learning of the correct technic more difficult.

Techniques of Tonsillectomy

Dissection

This is the technique we prefer. The patient should be positioned on the table with the head extended and the occiput lower than the shoulders. In

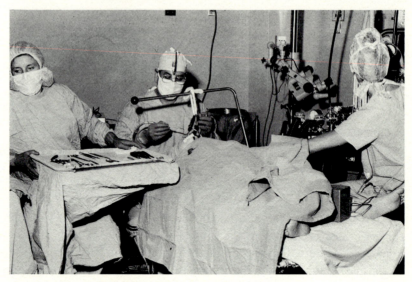

Fig. 1. Position of the patient and instruments for tonsillectomy.

this position, gravity causes any blood to pool in the nasopharynx. The operation is carried out under direct vision. The mucous membrane of the tonsillar pillars is incised and the upper pole is delivered exposing the smooth white capsule. The tonsil is dissected from the pharyngeal wall in this plane and finally the attachments of the lower pole are divided and the tonsil removed. The critical point of technic is the correct identification of the correct plane of dissection. It is here that the extra visibility afforded by the use of a suction dissector is most helpful.

Tonsillectomy by dissection can be used as an immediate definitive treatment of peritonsillar abscess [4].

Guillotine

The use of a tonsil guillotine depends on the fact that the tonsil capsule is not adherent to its bed and so can be dislocated from the pharyngeal wall. The great majority of children's tonsils can be removed by the guillotine technic. However, it is not so suitable for adults as after multiple attacks of tonsillitis or peritonsillar abscess, the capsule becomes adherent to the pharyngeal wall.

The main advantage of the guillotine is the speed of operation, but compared to dissection, guillotining is a blind procedure in which the tonsil is sheared out rather than dissected under vision. A disadvantage of the guillotine is that it often leaves the lower pole behind, and this tonsil remainant may hypertrophy to become indistinguishable from an untouched tonsil.

It takes considerable practice to acquire the knack of using a tonsil guillotine efficiently.

Cryosurgery

After 3–5 min freezing with a cryoprobe, a tonsil immediately becomes edematous. After 24 h a necrotic area appears and after 8–10 days, this gradually sloughs.

Cryosurgery has the advantage that patients can be treated as outpatients under local anesthesia. The cold itself produces anesthesia. Postoperative pain may be somewhat lessened and the risk of operative or postoperative bleeding is less. The major disadvantage is that large tonsillar remnants frequently occur after a single cryoprobe applications and multiple cryosurgical treatments may be necessary to achieve a complete tonsillectomy.

Miscellaneous

Tonsillectomy may be accomplished by electrocautery [6] or the use of caustic agents but these techniques are not in common use and appear to offer no particular advantages.

Radiation has no place in the treatment of inflammatory diseases of the tonsil, because of the risk of the patient later developing a neoplasm.

Techniques of Hemostasis after Tonsillectomy

Ligatures and electrocautery are both very effective methods of obtaining hemostasis.

Ligation

The bleeding vessel is picked up in a tonsil hemostat and a ligature applied. The use of a recurved hemostat of the Negus pattern makes tying this ligature much easier. Alternatively the ligature may be applied as a slip knot. This is the only place in surgical technique in which such a knot is justifiable [7]. A suture ligature can be passed in figure of eight fashion around the vessel and tied to control the hemorrhage.

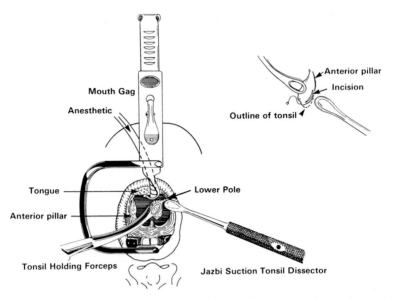

Fig. 2. Diagrammatic representation of suction tonsillectomy technique (see text for details).

Electrocautery

Either unipolar or bipolar cautery can be used to control hemorrhage. The use of insulated forceps to pick up the bleeding point makes this an easy method of hemostasis.

Packing

A tonsil sponge applied under pressure for a time will stop most minor bleeding. This is a useful way of controlling a generalized ooze. SELTZER [9] recommended the use of a special cellulose sponge which would expand in the tonsillar fossa.

Local Drugs

Epinephrine can be injected into the tonsillar bed when the operation is done under local anesthesia. This decreases intraoperative bleeding considerably.

Astringents such as silver nitrate or tannic acid have been applied to the tonsil bed. Tannic acid has the advantage that it makes bleeding points easily identifiable. The tannic acid stains the tonsil bed brown and the bleeding points stand out as red blood on the brown background.

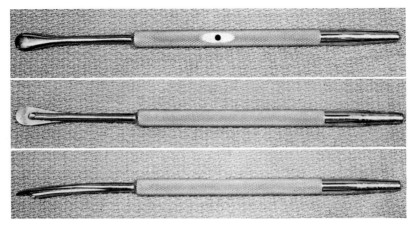

Fig. 3-5. Jazbi suction tonsil dissector.

Parenteral Medications

Premarin, adrenosem and epislon amino caproic acid have been tried to decrease the amount of bleeding associated with tonsillectomy [10]. None of these drugs have gained wide acceptance and the control of hemorrhage is primarily by techniques applied locally to the tonsillar bed.

Suction Tonsillectomy

The technique is not new, but a combination and modification of various techniques and instruments which we used during the course of our training and/or saw at the various University departments in different parts of the world.

The technique is simple. The tonsil is grasped with tonsil holding forceps and pulled medially to identify landmarks, especially the anterior pillar. A submucous incision is made near the upper pole, and extended around the pole and along the anterior and posterior pillars. The tonsil is dissected by peeling the tonsillar capsule away from the upper pole and the tonsillar bed, towards the lower pole where it is severed from the tongue by the dissector tip.

The biggest advantage of this technique is the relatively bloodless operative field due to readily available suction adjacent to the dissector. It needs only two basic instruments, a tonsil holder and the 'Jazbi suction tonsil dissector' (V. Mueller Instrument Company, Chicago, USA). The suction is controlled by the surgeon. This not only provides controlled suction, but also eliminates the need for an assistant or suction by a nurse or an anesthesiologist. The limited number of instruments used in this technique can easily be handled by the surgeon himself.

'Jazbi Suction Tonsil Dissector'

The dissector consists of two ends, one is connected to the suction tubing while the other, which is semicircular in shape, acts as a dissector. The tip of the dissector is sharp like a knife for incision and is serrated on one side for maximum sharpness. It can be used as a blunt dissector employing the serrated side of the instrument. The shaft of the instrument conceals a suction tubing, $^1/_8$ inch in diameter. It is adequate not only for fresh bleeding, but small blood clots as well. At the junction of anterior $^1/_3$ with the posterior $^2/_3$, there is an oval depression to support the thumb for better handling of the instrument and a hole for suction control. The instrument is approximately $7^1/_2$ inches long and weighes 40.5 g. It offers easy handling and maneuverability.

References

1 Workshop on Tonsillectomy and Adenoidectomy. Ann. Otol. Rhinol. Lar. *84:* suppl. 19, pp. 1–79 (1975).
2 PRATT, L. W.: Tonsillectomy and adenoidectomy morbidity and mortality. Trans. Am. Acad. Ophthal. Oto-lar. *75:* 1146–1154 (1974).
3 WILSON, T. G.: Diseases of the ear, nose, and throat in children, pp. 224–248 (Heinemann, London 1962).
4 YUNG, A. K. and CANTRELL, R. W.: Quinsy tonsillectomy. Laryngoscope *86:* 1714 to 1717 (1976).
5 SCHOUSBOE, H. H. and AASTRUP, J. E.: J. Lar. Otol. *90:* 795–799 (1976).
6 HOLLANDER, A. R.: Office practice otolaryngology (Davis, Philadelphia 1965).
7 LORE, J. M.: An atlas of head and neck surgery; vol. 2, 2nd ed. (Saunders, Philadelphia 1973).
8 RITTER, F. and JOSEPH, D.: Tonsillectomy and adenoidectomy. Panel discussions; Pediatric otolaryngology. Otol. Clin. N. Am. *10:* 247 (1977).
9 SELTZER, A. P.: Control of tonsillar hemorrhage. Use of a new cellulose material. J. nath. med. Ass. *61:* 333–334 (1969).
10 VERSTRAETE, M; VERMYLEN, J., and TYBERGHEIN, J.: Double blind evaluation of the hemostatic effect of adrenochrome monosemicarbazone, conjugated estrogens and epsilon amino caproic acid after adenotonsillectomy. Acta haemat. *40:* 154–161 (1968).

B. JAZBI, MD, DLO, FAAP, Professor and Chief of Otorhinolaryngology, University of Missouri, Kansas City, School of Medicine, The Children's Mercy Hospital, *Kansas City, MO 64108* (USA)

Adv. Oto-Rhino-Laryng., vol. 23, pp. 115–130 (Karger, Basel 1978)

Neoplasms of the Head and Neck in Children

James B. Snow, jr.

Department of Otorhinolaryngology and Human Communication,
University of Pennsylvania School of Medicine, Philadelphia, Pa.

Introduction

Important progress has been made in recent years in the diagnosis and treatment of children with neoplasms of the head and neck. The application of diagnostic techniques such as angiography in childhood neoplasms such as angiofibromas of the nasopharynx and computerized tomography in orbital neoplasms have resulted in more rational therapeutic approaches. The use of multiple modality therapy in highly lethal childhood neoplasms, such as Hodgkin's and non-Hodkin's lymphomas and rhabdomyosarcomas, has resulted in striking improvements in survival rates. The improvement in survival in Hodgkin's disease treated with extended field radiation and prolonged combination chemotherapy and in rhabomyosarcoma by the application of surgery to remove the bulk of the tumor, radiation therapy and combined and prolonged chemotherapy are most gratifying.

Malignant tumors in children are rare; however, cancer kills more children at the present time than does any other disease in the age group 1–14 years and is second to trauma as a cause of death in that age group [1]. 41 % of cancers in children are leukemia (31 %) and lymphoma (10 %); 27 % are sarcomas (soft tissue, 14 % and bone, 13 %); 16 % are embryonal tumors (neuroblastoma, 9 % and Wilms' tumor, 7 %); 6 % are neural tumors (retinoblastoma); 5 % are carcinomas and adenocarcinomas and all others comprise 5 % [2]. The overall incidence of cancer is 10.79 per 100,000 children per year [3]. Approximately 4,000 children die each year from cancer in the United Staates, and nearly 50 % of those deaths are due to leukemia [1, 4]. A striking difference exists between childhood and adult cancers in that carcinomas and adenocarcinomas are rare in children while they comprise the majority of malignant neoplasms in adults.

The vast majority of neoplasms of the head and neck in children are benign. These benign neoplasms are predominantly of mesodermal origin. Several of the benign neoplasms are life-threatening because of their location as, for example, squamous cell papillomas of the larynx or because of their behavior as in the juvenile nasopharyngeal angiofibroma. The benign neoplasms of the head and neck in children in order of frequency are: hemangiomas, lymphangiomas, papillomas, fibromas, neurofibromas, juvenile nasopharyngeal angiofibromas, craniopharyngiomas, dermoids, teratomas and nasal gliomas.

Benign Neoplasms

Hemangiomas of the head and neck in children present special problems and their behavior is unpredicable. The special problems stem from the cosmetic deformity of the face, head, and neck that they may produce; the threat to function and life that may result from their locations in the oral cavity, pharynx and larynx, bleeding secondary to ulceration of the overlying skin and mucous membrane particularly in the oral cavity and the trapping of platelets that occasionally occurs to produce thrombocytopenia purpura. The diagnosis is ordinarily based on the clinical findings, and biopsy as a general rule is not necessary or advisable. Extreme conservatism regarding surgery should be exercised in the management of children with hemangiomas. One of the major advances in this field is the recognition that these tumors respond to corticosteroid therapy. This fact does not mean that it is appropriate to treat all children with hemangiomas with corticosteroids. The usual behavior of hemangiomas in children is to grow with the child for a certain period, usually 18 months, and then to involute. Unless a hemangioma is trapping platelets, undergoing ulceration is a threat to the maintenance of nutrition or the airway, corticosteroids should usually be withheld. Therapy for cosmetic purposes *per se* is questionable. A hemangioma in the subglottic area produces inspiratory stridor and progressive upper airway obstruction. At direct laryngoscopy, it appears as a reddish purple subglottic mass. Biopsy is not required and indeed is inappropriate because of the risk of uncontrolled bleeding in the respiratory tract. In this instance, the indication for corticosteroid therapy is clear-cut and regularly results in a reduction in the size of the lesion [5].

Squamous cell papillomas occur throughout the upper respiratory tract in children. There is considerable evidence that they are of viral etiology.

Papillomas produce the greatest problem in the larynx. Many forms of therapy including topical podophyllin, prolonged systemic tetracycline, and vaccines, have failed to produce reliable control of papilloma. Transfer factor changes the gross and microscopic appearence of the papilloma and is one of the most promising lines of research in this problem [6]. Recently, levamisole, a veterinary antihelminthic, has appeared to be helpful in one patient[7]. Various forms of surgery remain the standard therapy. These have included ultrasonic radiation, cryosurgery, laser radiation and removal with forceps [8]. Care must be taken to avoid abrasion of normal tissue because of the likelihood of implanting the tumor. Specifically, tracheoscopy and bronchoscopy should be avoided unless there is a specific indication for them. Tracheotomy is usually required to insure an airway, and the papillomas must be removed periodically to maintain the voice and airway. The removal of the papillomas must be carried out gingerly to prevent trauma to the normal laryngeal structures so that when spontaneous involution of the papillomas occurs, the voice will be normal. Although radiation therapy is effective in the treatment of papillomas, it is specifically contraindicated because of the likelihood of radiation-induced carcinoma of the larynx 10–20 years later [9].

Juvenile angiofibromas of the nasopharynx occur predominantly in males during adolescence. These neoplasms arise from the vault and posterior wall of the nasopharynx and may invade the orbit and cranial cavity. A recent development is the delineation of the extent of the tumor by carotid angiography. The source of its blood supply can also be determined, and the vascular pattern on angiography is sufficiently specific to allow definitive management without a biopsy. The main blood supply to the neoplasm is usually the internal maxillary artery. Selective embolization of the major blood vessels supplying the neoplasm has been accomplished with an apparent reduction in blood loss at surgery [10]. There are a number of observations that this neoplasm decreases in size and vascularity on estrogen therapy. The transpalatal approach is the most widely used technique for removal of angiofibromas of the nasopharynx. Radiation therapy is the preferred treatment for patients with orbital or intracranial extension.

Craniopharyngiomas account for approximately 10 % of the intracranial neoplasms in children. Central nervous system neoplasms rank next to leukemia as a cause of death from neoplasms. Craniopharyngiomas are derived from Rathke's pouch and are composed of well-differentiated epithelial elements including ameloblasts, cysts and bone. The major portion of the neoplasm presents intracranially and produces visual field defects, extraocular muscle paralyses and hypopituitarism. Surgical decompression has been challenged as a form of treatment by radiation therapy [11]. The long-term survival rate with radiation therapy is 75–90 % and the residual defects tend to be minimal.

Dermoids and teratomas occur in the head and neck in children, and their most common site in the head and neck is the nasopharynx [12]. Calcification in teratomas may be demonstrated on lateral radiographs of the nasopharynx and neck. Death can result from airway obstruction. The obstruction can usually be relieved with an oral airway. Surgical removal must be carefully planned to insure an adequate airway preoperatively, intra-operatively, and postoperatively. Although a tracheotomy is not usually necessary, it may be required in certain patients. Generally, endotracheal intubation for general anesthesia has allowed the successful transoral re-moval of the pedunculated tumors. More sessile tumors may require a trans-palatal approach.

Nasal gliomas are usually apparent at birth on the dorsum of the nose, and they have intranasal components and not infrequently intracranial con-nections. Excision of the nasal components should be preceded by a frontal craniotomy to exclude an intracranial connection [13].

Malignant Neoplasms

Major advances have occurred in the treatment of children with lym-phomas, rhabdomyosarcomas, and mucoepidermoid carcinomas of the salivary glands. The management of children with malignant neoplasms requires close cooperation among pediatric medical oncologists, radiation therapists, head and neck surgeons, diagnostic radiologists, pathologists, psychologists, social workers, nurses, speech pathologists, and prosthedon-tists. These advances have resulted primarily from the imaginative appli-cation of multiple modalities of therapy including chemotherapy, radiation therapy and surgery as well as the application of new diagnostic and staging techniques to define the extent of the tumor at the onset of therapy.

The radical surgery that is currently appropriate for adults with malig-nant neoplasms of the head and neck is less appropriate in children. In con-trast to the situation in adults, many malignant neoplasms in children are quite responsive to chemotherapy and radiation therapy and they may be used to convert inoperable neoplasms to operable ones or, depending on the sequence of therapy, surgery that does not completely remove the tumor may be adequate for successful treatment in combination with postoperative radiation therapy or chemotherapy. In general, two strategies can be used from the surgeon's point of view. The tumor may be wounded by a combination of radiation therapy and chemotherapy, and the surgery can be performed to remove the remaining neoplasm or the surgery can be carried out first to attempt to remove all or at least the bulk of the neoplasm and to follow the excision with tumorcidal radiation therapy combined with prolonged chemotherapy. The latter strategy has been used more extensively, and there are a number of specific neoplasms in which this strategy has been demonstrated to be highly effective. In addition to these documented advances in multimodal therapy, radical surgery currently appropriate to the adult should be tempered by the consequences of deforming surgery in the growing child which are more profound physically and psychologically than in the adult. The technical ability to resect extensive involvement of functionally and cosmetically important tissue in the head and neck is no less in the child than it is in the adult, but it must be modulated with the effects of such surgery on a child and with the now apparent good results of more limited resections in combination with radiation therapy and chemotherapy. Nevertheless, it is important for the operation to be as adequate a cancer operation as possible with attention to en bloc resection, wide surgical margins and special attention to possible perineural and intravascular extension.

Lymphoma

Hodgkin's disease is a distinct entity from the other lymphomatous diseases and occurs with sufficient frequency to merit consideration in the differential diagnosis of neck masses in children. It is extremely rare before 5 years of age. The peak incidence is in the 5- to 9-year age group. There is a three to one male predominance [14]. Painless lymphadenopathy in the lower part of the neck with or without fever is the most common presenting complaint. Anorexia, malaise, and weight loss are often present. Lymphadenopathy in the axilla and inguinal areas as well as hepatomegaly and splenomegaly may be present. Chest X-rays for mediastinal and hilar nodes are helpful, and lymphangiography is used to demonstrate retroperitoneal involvement. Bone marrow biopsies rarely demonstrate Reed-Sternberg cells.

The biopsy of neck nodes is frequently useful in diagnosis. A whole

lymph node with minimum trauma to it gives the pathologist the best opportunity to arrive at a correct diagnosis. An enlarging node low in the neck is
most likely to yield the diagnosis of Hodgkin's disease.

Accurate staging allows rational planning of therapy and has been
credited as a major factor in the dramatic improvement in survival rates.
Stage I is lymphadenopathy limited to one lymphatic region. Stages I through
IV are further subdivided on the basis of whether there are constitutional
signs such as fever into A, with no constitutional symptoms, and B, with
constitutional symptoms. Stage II is disease limited to one side of the diaphragm. Stage III is involvement of lymphatic systems on both sides of the
diaphragm, and stage IV is dissemination to involve lung, liver, bone marrow, shin and central nervous system.

Laparotomy is used in many centers for staging and provides delineation
of splenic, hepatic, and retroperitoneal node involvement and the opportunity for splenectomy. Involved lymph nodes at the splenic hilus can be
detected, and splenectomized patients seem to tolerate radiation therapy
and chemotherapy better but are subject to life-threatening infections and
small bowel obstruction from adhesions.

Radiation therapy is the treatment of choice for patients with stage I
and II Hodgkin's disease. KAPLAN [15] has reported progressive improvement
in survival rates over the last 30 years with a 73.3 % 5-year survival with
6 Mew linear accelerator radiation therapy.

In patients whose diagnosis is established with excisional biopsy of a
cervical lymph node, the neck and mediastinum are treated. Permanent
control has been reported with 3,000 rad given in 3 weeks from cobalt-60 or
other appropriate megavoltage sources. Combination chemotherapy and
radiation therapy for patients with stage III and IV Hodgkin's disease achieve
remission in 70–80 %; and of the patients achieving remission, 80 % survive
for 5 years and 40 % are disease-free. The chemotherapy for patient with
Hodgkin's disease consists of intensive, intermittent therapy programs referred to as combination chemotherapy, such as the MOPP protocol which
employs 14–day cycles with nitrogen mustard, 6 mg/m^2 intravenously on
days 1 and 8, vincristine 1.4 mg/m^2 intravenously on days 1 and 8, procarbazine 100 mg/m^2 orally for 14 days and prednisone 40 mg/m^2 orally for
14 days in cycles 1 and 4 only. Rest periods of 14 days are allowed between
cycles [16].

The principles of combination chemotherapy include the use of several
agents with differing toxicities for additive or even synergistic antitumor
effects without prohibitive toxicity. Chemotherapeutic agents are classified

according to their activity or origin as: alkylating agents (nitrogen mustard, busulphan, chlorambucil, cyclophosphamide, bischloroethylnitrosourea [BCNU], chloroethylcyclohexylnitrosurea [CCNU]; antimetabolites (6-mercaptopurine, methotrexate, fluorouracil, cytosine arabinoside, and thioguanine); antibiotics (actinomycin D, mitomycin C, methromycin, daunorubicin, streptozocin, bleomycin and adriamycin); plant extracts (vincristine, vinblastine and podophyllin); enzymes (L-asparaginase and zanthinoxidase); steroids (corticosteroids, androgens, and estrogens), and miscellaneous agents such as procarbazine (methylhydrazine), hydroxycarbamide (hydroxyurea), and dimethyl-triazino-imidazole carboxamide (DTIC).

Mitosis is followed by an interval, G_1, after wich a period of DNA synthesis called the S phase leads to the premitotic G_2 phase after which mitosis occurs. Cells not passing through a cycle after mitosis are in the G_0 phase. Chemotherapeutic agents can also be categorized as to their effect relative to cell kinetics (cell division) as phase-specific agents (vincristine, vinblastine, bleomycin, methotrexate, 6-mercaptopurine, cytosine arabinoside, hydroxyurea, BCNU, CCNU, and DTIC), cycle specific agents (cyclophosphamide, fluorouracil, actinomycin D, daunorubicin, mitomycin C, and adriamycin) and nonspecific agents (nitrogen mustard, mitomycin C, DTIC, BCNU, and CCNU). In leukemia, certain agents are more suitable for induction of remission (prednisone and vincristine), maintenance of remission (methotrexate and 6-mercaptopurine) and reinduction during remission. In solid tumors these concepts are less well defined.

Sequential administration of nonspecific drugs like alkylating agents followed by cycle-specific and phase-specific agents would appear rational providing agents with quantitatively different mechanisms and toxicities are given and time is given to allow vital normal stem cells to return to a mainly nonproliferating state.

In a recent report, the 5-year survival rates for children with Hodgkin's disease increased from 50% in 1964 to 73% in 1968 to 95% in 1973. This improvement was attributed to sequential introduction of lymphangiography and laparotomy with splenectomy, the change from involved field to extended field radiation and the introduction of multiple agent chemotherapy at first for relapse and more recently as elective initial therapy combined with extended field radiation for children in advanced stages [17].

In patients with stage III and IV disease, two courses of MOPP precede radiotherapy. Depending on the clinical situation, the mediastinum, abdomen, pelvis, and peripheral nodal areas are radiated in sequence. In the usual case, the lower torso receives radiation followed by a 4- to 8-week rest period for hematopoietic recovery. Radiation therapy to the pelvis and mediastinum and neck is then given.

The non-Hodgkin's lymphomas that occur in children are undifferentiated lymphoma of the Burkitt's type, undifferentiated lymphoma of the non-Burkitt's type and histiocyctic lymphoma (histiocyctic reticulum cell sarcoma). In this nomenclature, undifferentiated means not nodular and not lymphocytic, types that occur in adults but not in children [18]. It would be well to delete the term lymphosarcoma in pediatric oncology. These three types of non-Hodgkin's lymphoma can be differentiated histopathologically and have unique clinical patterns.

Burkitt's lymphoma occurs in the jaws and abdominal viscera of African children [19]. It accounts for 50% of the malignant neoplasms in African children, but only 6–10% of lymphomas in children elsewhere. The male predominance is approximately five to one, and the peak incidence is from 5 to 9 years of age. In Africa, where the annual rainfall exceeds 20 inches and the mean temperature remains above 60 °F, the jaw and abdominal presentation of Burkitt's lymphoma occurs. The maxilla is involved three times more frequently than the lower jaw. Approximately one third of the children with the African presentation have abdominal involvement. In the form of the disease seen in North America, abdominal pain, nausea, and vomiting occur in 65%, mass in the jaws in 20%, cervical mass in 15%, and serous peritoneal or pleural effusions in 30% [20]. In contrast to the African variety, the male:female ratio is 1.3:1 and constitutional findings of fever, anoxia, and weight loss are usual.

The work-up is the same as for Hodgkin's disease. For the African presentation staging is as follows: stage I, single facial mass; stage II, two or more facial masses; stage III, intrathoracic, intra-abdominal, paraspinal or osseous masses; and stage IV, central nervous system or bone marrow involvement. The relative infrequency of facial involvement in the American presentation precludes the use of this staging system.

The prognosis of patients with Burkitt's lymphoma has undergone the most remarkable change in 15 years. Burkitt's lymphoma could not be treated successfully with radiation therapy. In 1961, the mean survival time was 6–12 weeks [21]. Now with multiple drug therapy (methotrexate and cyclophosphamide) 80% of stage I and stage II patients have long-term remissions and perhaps cures and at least 30% of children in all stages become free of the disease for long periods [22]. Cyclophosphamide is the therapy of choice in Burkitt's lymphoma.

Non-Burkitt's lymphoma rarely involves the head and neck. It tends to undergo leukemic transformation. The staging is the same as with Hodgkin's disease. Combination radiation therapy and chemotherapy regimens are usually employed, but no consistently effective chemotherapeutic protocol has been developed.

Histocystic lymphoma is rare and clinically ill-defined. It involves the oral structures and cervical lymph nodes. Radiation therapy and chemotherapy are used in treatment, but no successful treatment protocol has been established.

Sarcoma

Rhabdomyosarcomas are the most common soft tissue sarcomas in children. Fibrosarcomas, liposarcomas, leiomyosarcomas, hemangiopericytomas, and hemangioendotheliomas (angiosarcomas) rarely occur in the head and neck in children.

The most common sites for rhabdomyoscarcomas are in the head and neck. 30–60% occur in the head and neck, and 30% of those that arise in the head and neck occur in the orbit. They occur in the ear, nose, nasopharynx, maxilla, oral cavity, pharynx, larynx, soft tissues of the face as well as elsewhere in the body. Rhabdomyosarcomas of the head and neck metastasize to the cervical lymph nodes.

In the past, the survival rate ranged from 20 to 25% with radical surgery. The prognosis for patients with orbital lesions undergoing exenteration of the orbital contents was better and approximated 50% 5-year survival. The prognosis for all patients with rhabdomyosarcoma has changed dramatically for the better, and patients with rhabdomyosarcoma of the head and neck share in this improved outlook. Surgical removal of the bulk of the lesion, radiation therapy and combination chemotherapy with vincristine, actinomycin D, and cyclophosphamide in patients with head and neck rhabdomyosarcomas have resulted in 74% (14 of 19 patients) achieving a neoplasm free status for 3–10 years with a mean of 3.7 years [23]. In another series of 29 patients, 24 (20 stage I and II and 4 stage III) or 82% are alive and without evidence of tumor 4–42 months after completion of treatment [24]. Some advocate radiation therapy and chemotherapy without orbital exenteration for orbital rhabdomyosarcomas and demonstrate a 70% 5-year survival without exenteration of the orbit. The most widely employed treatment plans for head and neck rhabdomyosarcomas consist of initial resection of the tumor. If the margins are free of tumor, chemotherapy is initiated and continued for 2 years. If the lesion cannot be removed or if the margins of the resection are not microscopically free of tumor, radiation therapy is given to a dose of 5,000–6,000 rad in a 5- to 6-week period. Actinomycin D is given at the onset of the radiation therapy and 2 mg/m² (max 2 mg) are given weekly for 12 weeks. At the end of the radiation therapy, cyclophosphamide is given 2.5 mg/kg p.o. daily for 2 years.

Fibrosarcoma and neurofibrosarcoma have a predilection in children for the head and neck, and 25% of them occur in these anatomical areas. Fibrosarcomas and neurofibrosarcomas are the next most common tumor of the head and neck in children after rhabdomyosarcomas. They occur in the neck, cheek, mandible, nose and pharynx. There is a two to one male predominance. The main problem is the tendency toward local recurrence after excision, and metastasis is rare. Neurofibrosarcomas occurring near the base of the skull are often dumbbell shaped with intracranial as well as extracranial masses. This problem could be demonstrated by computerized tomography. No generally accepted treatment plan exists. Radiation therapy to 6,000 rad in combination with actinomycin D therapy preoperative to radical resection appears to be a rational approach to rare sarcomas that are only moderately sensitive to radiation therapy and often recur after radical resection. The strategy in this instance is to wound the tumor with radiation therapy and chemotherapy before proceeding with radical resection. A similar strategy can be applied to patients with liposarcomas, leiomyosarcomas, hemangiopericytomas, and angiosarcomas.

Osteogenic sarcoma of the head and neck is fortunately rare, but it does occur in the lower jaw and very unusually in the maxilla. There are no statistics limited to patients with head and neck osteogenic sarcomas. Jaffe et al. [25] have demonstrated that the incidence of metastasis was significantly reduced in patients who received vincristine and methotrexate after surgery and radiation. Pulmonary metastasis has regressed in 4 of 10 patients on chemotherapy [26].

Ewing's sarcoma is as likely to occur in children as in the older age group. Approximately 5% of those occurring in children are in the head and neck. The current theory is that Ewing's sarcoma is a myelogenous neoplasm similar to a plasma cell myeloma. It characteristically is multicentric in several bones at one time. The skull bones, maxilla, mandible, and cervical vertebrae may be involved. Encouraging results have been reported with Ewing's sarcoma. Hustu et al. [27] reported complete regression of tumor in 66% of their patients for 4–91 months with combination radiotherapy and chemotherapy with cyclophosphamide and vincristine. With the addition of actinomycin D even better results have been reported. Rosen et al. [28]

reported 12 children in disease-free remission 10–37 months after radiation therapy and sequential adjuvant chemotherapy with actinomycin D, adriamycin, vincristine and cyclophosphamide.

Neuroblastomas

Neuroblastomas are embryonal neoplasms like Wilms' tumors and appear early in childhood. Neuroblastomas occur as fairly well differentiated ganglioneuromas and ganglioneuroblastomas, poorly differentiated sympathicoblastomas and in a special variety, olfactory neuroesthesiomas. Characteristically, neuroblastomas arise from neural crest tissue along the distribution of the sympathetic chain including the cranial ganglia and the adrenal medulla. These neoplasms secrete varying amounts of catecholamines. Neuroblastomas are one of the most common malignant neoplasms in children, but only 7% of them arise primarily in the head and neck; 2% arise in the head and 5% arise in the neck. These neoplasms arising from the cervical sympathetic ganglia often produce cranial nerve palsies, extend through the intervertebral foramina, and compress the spinal cord or may extend into the cranial cavity through the foramina of the base of the skull. Neuroblastomas metastasize early and may metastasize to the head and neck from other areas. Metastases are not as likely to produce neurologic symptoms and signs because the metastasis is usually to lymph nodes [29]. Metastasis to the mandible occurs from distant sites. There is a predilection for skeletal metastases, and the lung parenchyma is spared.

Calcification in the neoplasm frequently gives it a speckled appearance radiographically. Skeletal survey, 24-hour collection of urine for catecholamines and bone marrow biopsy are required in the work-up of children suspected of having neuroblastomas.

Resection remains the treatment of choice. Neuroblastomas are responsive to radiation therapy and to vincristine and cyclophosphamide, but multimodal therapy has not enhanced the survival rate over that obtained with surgery alone as has occurred with rhabdomyosarcomas. The cure rate in surgically accessible lesions approaches 90%.

Olfactory neuroesthesiomas arise from the olfactory epithelium and differ in malignant potentiality from other neuroblastomas. They tend to recur following excision, but respond well to radiation therapy. The role of chemotherapy in the management of olfactory neuroesthesiomas has not been established.

Retinoblastomas

Retinoblastomas are rare hereditary malignant tumors. Two thirds of them are unilateral. They may be multicentric. The mode of transmission is by an autosomal dominant gene [30]. Retinoblastomas are malignant gliomas which invade the optic nerve and spread intracranially through the optic foramen. They cause a white pupil which is often first seen by the parents. Children in a retinoblastoma family should be followed with frequent eye examinations from birth. Enucleation with excision of 10–14 mm of optic nerve is the treatment of choice for unilateral neoplasms. The overall survival rate is 85 %. With bilateral neoplasms or a neoplasm in the remaining eye, radiation therapy is the treatment of choice and quite effective. Several chemotherapeutic agents are effective against the neoplasm including triethylene melamine (TEM), combined vincristine and cyclophosphamide and combined actinomycin D, chlorambucil and methotrexate, but the results of treatment for central nervous system spread and distant metastasis are disappointing.

Carcinoma

Carcinoma in the head and neck in children is rare. It occurs in the salivary glands, particularly the parotid gland, the nasopharynx and the thyroid gland.

Carcinomas of the salivary glands in children are predominantly of the mucoepidermoid type [31]. Malignant mixed tumors, adenoid cystic carcinomas, adenocarcinomas and undifferentiated carcinoma also occur in children [32]. Mucoepidermoid carcinomas are treated by parotidectomy with sparing of the facial nerve if compatible with complete excision. Whether or not a radical neck dissection should be carried out depends on whether the mucoepidermoid carcinoma is high grade or low grade. The high grade lesions are more likely to metastasize, and a radical neck dissection should be performed in patients with them [33]. Patients with malignant mixed tumors and adenoid cystic carcinomas should be treated with parotidectomy. Patients with adenocarcinomas require parotidectomy and radical neck dissection as do patients with the rare undifferentiated carcinomas.

Carcinoma of the nasopharynx occurs in children with the histopathologic picture designated as lymphoepithelioma in which anaplastic epithelial cells are surrounded by normal appearing lymphoid cells [34]. Metastasis to cervical lymph nodes occurs early in carcinoma of the nasopharynx. Distant metastasis becomes clinically evident late. The treatment of carcinoma of the nasopharynx in children is radiation therapy as it is in adults. The radiation therapy should be delivered to both sides of the neck whether there are clinically demonstrated metastases or not. A total tumor dose of 7,000 rad should be delivered to the primary and 5,000 rad to each side of the neck. Surgery plays no role in the initial therapy of carcinoma of the nasopharynx. Those cervical metastases that remain clinically palpable after radiation therapy or that subsequently become apparent should be eradicated by radical neck dissection [35]. The role of chemotherapy for carcinoma of the nasopharynx in children has not been determined.

Immunologic similarities exist in patients with Burkitt's lymphoma, nasopharyngeal carcinoma, and infectious mononucleosis. The Epstein-Barr virus (EBV) is the etiologic factor in infectious mononucleosis. The EBV was originally isolated from cultured cell lines from patients with Burkitt's lymphoma. Elevated titers of anti-EBV antibodies have been found in patients with Burkitt's lymphoma and nasopharyngeal carcinoma [36]. Although significantly high antibody titers to EBV are present in only 45 % of stage I carcinoma of the nasopharynx, the titers are elevated in 100 % of patients with stage V lesions [37]. Treated patients without evidence of persistent neoplasm have lower titers. The role of the EBV in the etiology of Burkitt's lymphoma and carcinoma of the nasopharynx is obscured by the fact that the virus can persist in lymphoid tissue for long periods as a latent infection. Therefore, its presence in these diseases may be on the basis of a previous EBV infection. Although the EBV may not be the etiologic agent in Burkitt's lymphoma and carcinoma of the nasopharynx, it appears to be a necessary factor for Burkitt's lymphoma and carcinoma of the naso-pharynx. There is apparently some other unidentified necessary factor.

Thyroid carcinoma occurs occasionally in children and may be of the medullary, papillary and mixed papillary and follicular types. The papillary and mixed papillary and follicular types are more common. The medullary form is less common and may occur as an autosomal dominant hereditary disease associated with pheochromocytomas and neuromas. There is a two to one female predominance for carcinoma of the thyroid in children. A total thyroidectomy is the treatment of choice if there are no palpable nodes. If there are palpable nodes, a modified radical neck dissection with preservation of the spinal accessory nerve and sternocleidomastoid muscle may be carried out in continuity with the total thyroidectomy. Thyroid hormone should be given to reduce thyrotoxin secretion to eliminate the stimulus for further growth of any residual neoplasm. Radioactive iodine may be used in the presence of recurrent neoplasm. The disease is relatively benign in children, but unfortunately variable. A fatal outcome occurs in a number of patients. The offspring of patients with medullary carcinoma of the thyroid should be screened for medullary carcinoma with calcitonin determinations.

Malignant melanomas are relatively rare in children, but when they do occur there is a predilection for the head and neck. 60% occur in the head and neck and they are usually pigmented although amelanotic melanomas do occur. Wide surgical excision with approximately 5-cm margins and radical neck dissection is the treatment of choice. The behavior of melanomas in children is similar to that in adults, and the principles of therapy are the same in the two age groups [38].

Radical resection of neoplasms of the head and neck in children pose complex, cosmetic and psychological difficulties to the child and parent. Although cure in the pediatric age group often depends on a combination of surgery, irradiation and chemotherapy, the surgery has a critical role. If the parents can accept the problems presented, then the child usually will. Gratifying resumption of normal life pattern can follow partial maxillectomy in the child. Although it is the wrong philosophy to be as radical in the child as is customarily practiced in adult head and neck oncology, it is likewise wrong to be unwilling to carry out the surgery necessary to obtain the gratifying results now available in many malignant neoplasms of the head and neck in children.

References

1   American Cancer Society '72 Cancer Facts and Figures 1972, The Society.
2   Sutow, W.W.: Drug therapy and curability of childhood cancer. Postgrad. Med. 48: 173–177 (1970).
3   Sutow, W.W.; Vietti, T.J., and Fernbach, D.J. (eds): Clinical pediatric oncology, p. 2 (Mosby, Louis 1973).
4   Miller, R.W.: Fifty-two forms of childhood cancer; United States Mortality Experience, 1960–1966. J. Pediat. 75: 685–689 (1969).
5   Cohen, S.R. and Wang, C.I.: Steroid treatment of hemangioma of the head and neck in children. Ann. Otol. Rhinol. Lar. 81: 584–590 (1972).
6   Quick, C.A.; Behrens, H.W.; Brinton-Darnell, M., and Good, R.A.: Treatment of papillomatosis of the larynx with transfer factor. Ann. Otol. Rhinol. Lar. 84: 607–613 (1975).
7   Rosa, E. de: Laryngeal papilloma, new treatment with levamisole. Trans. Am. Acad. Ophthal. Otol. 84: 75–77 (1977).

8   STRONG, M.S. and JAKO, G.J.: Laser surgery in the larynx early clinical experience
    with continuous CO_2 laser. Ann. Otol. Rhinol. Lar. *81:* 791–798 (1972).

9   RABBETT, W.F.: Juvenile laryngeal papillomatosis. The relationship of irradiation
    to malignant degeneration in the disease. Ann. Otol. Rhinol. Lar. *74:* 1149–1163
    (1965).

10 BILLER, H.F.; SESSIONS, D.G., and OGURA, J.H.: Angiofibroma: a treatment
    approach. Laryngoscope *84:* 695–706 (1974).

11 KRAMER, S.: Radiation therapy in the management of brain tumors in children. Ann.
    N.Y. Acad. Sci. *159:* 571–584 (1969).

12 FELDER, H.: Benign congenital neoplasms: dermoids and teratomas. Archs Otolar.
    101: 333–334 (1975).

13 WALKER, E.A. and RESLER, D.R.: Nasal glioma. Laryngoscope *73:* 93–107 (1963).

14 SULLIVAN, M.P.; FULLER, L.M., and BUTLER, J.J.: Hodgkin's disease in children;
    in SUTOW *et al.* Clinical pediatric oncology (Mosby, St. Louis 1973).

15 KAPLAN, H.S.: Radiotherapy of advanced Hodgkin's disease with curative intent.
    J. Am. med. Ass. *233:* 52–54 (1973).

16 DEVITA, V.T.; SERPICK, A.A., and CARBONE, P.P.: Combination chemotherapy in
    the treatment of advanced Hodgkin's disease. Ann. Int. Med. *73:* 881–895 (1970).

17 JENKIN, R.D.T.; BROWN, T.C.; PETERS, M.V., and SONLEY, M.J.: Hodgkin's disease
    in children, a retrospective analysis 1958–73. Cancer *35:* 979–990 (1975).

18 SULLIVAN, M.P.: Non-Hodgkin's lymphoma of childhood; in SUTOW *et al.* Clinical
    pediatric oncology (Mosby, St. Louis 1973).

19 BURKITT, D.: A sarcoma involving the jaws of African children. Br. J. Surg. *46:*
    218–223 (1958).

20 COHEN, M.H.; BENNETT, J.M.; BERARD, C.W.; ZIEGLER, J.L.; VOGEL, C.L.;
    SHEAGREN, J.N., and CARBONE, P.P.: Burkitt's tumor in the United States. Cancer
    23: 1259–1272 (1969).

21 CLIFFORD, P.: Malignant disease of the nose, paranasal sinuses and post-nasal
    space in East Africa. J. Lar. Otol. *75:* 707–733 (1961).

22 CLIFFORD, P.: Prospectives in head and neck oncology. J. Lar. Otol. *90:* 221–251
    (1976).

23 DONALDSON, S.S.; CASTRO, J.R.; WILBUR, J.R., and JESSE, R.H.: Rhabdomyo-
    sarcoma of head and neck in children combination treatment by surgery, irradiation
    and chemotherapy. Cancer *31:* 26–35 (1973).

24 GHAVINI, F.; EXELBY, P.R.; D'ANGIO, G.J.; CHAM, W.; LIEBERMAN, P.H.; TAN, C.;
    MIKE, V., and MURPHY, M.L.: Multidisciplinary treatment of embryonal rhab-
    domyosarcoma in children. Cancer *35:* 677–686 (1975).

25 JAFFE, N.; FREI, E.; TRAGGIS, D., and BISHOP, Y.: Adjuvant methotrexate and
    citrovorum-factor treatment of osteogenic sarcoma. New Engl. J. Med. *291:* 994–997
    (1974).

26 JAFFE N. and PIED, D.: Recent advances in chemotherapy of metastatic osteogenic
    sarcoma. Cancer *30:* 1627–1630 (1972).

27 HUSTU, H.O.; PINKEL, D., and PRATT, C.B.: Treatment of clinically localized
    Ewing's sarcoma with radiotherapy and combined chemotherapy. Cancer *30:* 1522
    to 1527 (1972).

28 ROSEN, G.; WOLLNER, N.; TAN, C.; WU, S.J.; HAJDU, S.I.; CHAM, W.; D'ANGIO,
    G.J., and MURPHY, M.L.: Disease free survival in children with Ewing's sarcoma

treated with radiation therapy and adjuvant four drugs sequential chemotherapy. Cancer *33:* 384–393 (1974).

29   JAFFE, B.F. and JAFFE, N.: Diagnosis and treatment head and neck tumors in children. Pediatrics *51:* 731–740 (1973).

30   ELLSWORTH, R.M.: The practical management of retinoblastoma. Trans.Am. Ophthal.Soc. *67:* 462–534 (1969).

31   BAUM, R.K. and PERZIK, S.L.: Tumors of the parotid gland in children. Review of 40 cases. Am.Surg. *31:* 719–722 (1965).

32   GALICH, R.: Salivary gland neoplasms in childhood. Archs Otolar. *89:* 878–882 (1969).

33   HEALEY, W.V.; PERZIN, K.H., and SMITH, L.: Mucoepidermoid carcinoma of salivary gland origin. Cancer *26:* 368–388 (1970).

34   PICK, T.; MAURER, H.M., and McWILLIAMS, N.B.: Lymphoepithelioma in childhood. J.Pediat. *84:* 96–100 (1974).

35   SNOW, J.B.: Carcinoma of the nasopharynx in children. Ann.Otol.Rhinol.Lar. *84:* 817–827 (1975).

36   KLEIN, G.; GEERING, G.; OLD, L.J., *et al.:* Comparison of the anti-EBV titre and the EBV- associated membrane radioactive and precipitating antibody in the sera of Burkitts' lymphoma and nasopharyngeal carcinoma patients and controls. Int.J. Cancer *5:* 185–194 (1970).

37   HENLE, W.: Elevated antibody titers to Epstein-Barr virus in nasopharyngeal carcinoma, other head and neck neoplasms and control groups. J.natn.Cancer Inst. *44:* 225–231 (1970).

38   SHANON, E.; SAMUEL, Y.; ADLER, A.; RAPOPORT, Y., and REDIANU, C.: Malignant melanoma of the head and neck in children. Archs Otolar. *102:* 224–247 (1976).

J.B.SNOW, jr., MD, Professor and Chairman, Department of Otorhinolaryngology and Human Communication, University of Pennsylvania School of Medicine, *Philadelphia, Pa.* (USA)

Adv. Oto-Rhino-Laryng., vol. 23, pp. 131–154 (Karger, Basel 1978)

Maxillofacial Clefts

LESLIE BERNSTEIN

Department of Otorhinolaryngology, University of California, Davis, Calif.

The overall incidence of maxillofacial clefts ranges from 1:500 to 1:700 births. Where a history of clefts exists in the family, the incidence is much higher. In recent years, because of the ready availability of birth-control measures and genetic counseling, the incidence of these clefts has dropped somewhat.

Much progress has been made in the management of maxillofacial clefts over the past 30 years, various disciplines having made their individual contributions to the overall welfare of these unfortunate individuals. Consequently, it is usually possible to assure the parents of a newborn cleft lip and palate infant that, with time and with the proper management, the child should become an acceptable member of society, both with regard to esthetics and function.

The complexity of the deformity which is involved in maxillofacial clefts necessitates a multidisciplinary approach to its rehabilitation. In most cases, the treatment may extend over a span of 18 years – from birth until the final secondary esthetic operation – and even for life in some instances, as when obturators form part of the management. Yet, in spite of the vast progress that has been made, many modifications in the treatment are still being introduced, because results are as yet far from ideal. A new technique requires several years before its results may be adequately assessed. The accumulation of data and the need for long-term follow-up are thus very necessary. It is therefore important that maxillofacial cleft patients be treated in special centers where the services of a team of specialists are available and where the end-results of management may be critically evaluated.

Early Management
Emergency Treatment

The syndrome of cleft palate, micrognathia, and glossoptosis (commonly known as Robin's syndrome, although it was first described by FAIRBAIRN in 1846 [11]) may present as a neonatal respiratory emergency. To overcome blockage of the pharynx by the tongue that cannot be accommodated within the small mandibular arch, the tongue needs to be displaced forward. One way of achieving this is to suture it into the mandibular labial sulcus, where it is kept for several months until the mandible has reached normal proportions. This operation, first described by SHUKOWSKY in 1910 [11] and then reintroduced by DOUGLAS [9] in 1946, has proved very adequate in the management of such cases. Postoperatively, the mandible grows rather rapidly, reaching normal proportions within 6–12 months.

Counseling of Parents

Early psychologic counseling of the parents is of utmost importance. It is difficult to imagine the shock of parents, who have been expecting a perfectly normal baby, when they are confronted with what must appear to them as a gross monstrosity. The need for reassurance is not only humanitarian, but mandatory. It is important that the parents be told that proper management over the years will rehabilitate their child into a well-functioning and esthetically acceptable member of society. Frankness as to our ignorance of the cause of the deformity is necessary to avoid a sense of guilt in the parents, a situation which may seriously interfere with rehabilitation later on. The confidence and cooperation of the parents is essential in the long-term management which the majority of these patients require. An explanation of the deformity and an outline of the proposed treatment will enable the parents to better appreciate the problems involved in the overall management of their child.

It is also the surgeon's moral duty to explain the effect of heredity in these malformations. When such a hereditary link is obvious, the parents may well be advised to adopt additional children.

Feeding

Early management of cleft palate infants is primarily concerned with proper methods of feeding. Breast feeding is quite impractical and should not be attempted. A very satisfactory way of overcoming nasal regurgitation is to place the child in a lateral sloping position and to deposit the formula in the buccal cavity by means of a rubber syringe. Another useful means for introducing nourishment is the restaurant-type plastic ketchup dispenser. This is equipped with a small nozzle which can dispense formula in desired amounts when the bottle is gently squeezed. Feeding may also be accomplished with a rubber nipple that has had its hole enlarged. After boiling, such a nipple responds well to the gentle pressure of the tongue and the child is able to suck without fatigue.

In all cleft palate infants, feeding must be slow to allow sufficient time for swallowing. Because of the increased amount of air that is ingested in this manner, burping should be more frequent than with a normal infant. It is notable that when the parents participate in the feeding and in the care of the infant, they develop a deeper appreciation of the problems confronting the surgeon. Invariably, after the lip has been repaired, a more genuine acceptance develops and the physician finds that he is dealing with a happier family.

Maxillary Orthopedics

Widely separated, or poorly aligned, maxillary segments may be repositioned by means of removable prosthetic appliances, a technique known as maxillary orthopedics. Since repair of the cleft lip will reconstruct the labial muscular sphincter, which in turn will approximate the alveolar segments anteriorly, it is desirable that these segments be in proper alignment prior to this operation.

The services of a dental specialist (an orthodontist or a prosthodontist) who is familiar with such techniques, are necessary for this part of the management. The appliance is made in sections, corresponding to the cleft segments, and are joined together by a reciprocating screw, or screws. By this means, the separate segments of the appliance may be moved closer together, or spread wider apart, as necessary (fig. 1). Another variety, althoug in a single piece, is actually made of the component parts of the cleft. These are fused together in a progressively favorable position at intervals of days or weeks. By sucking on the appliance, the infant promotes the gentle repositioning of the segments.

Reapproximation of the maxillary segments simultaneously advances the lateral lip segments closer together, thus facilitating the lip repair. In instances of bilateral clefts of the palate, where the premaxilla may be somewhat protrusive, maxillary orthopedics may reduce the distance between the segments to allow closure of the bilateral cleft lip with little tension. A fringe benefit of these orthopedic appliances is that they aid the infant in feeding. It is remarkable that, when the appliance is removed, the infant will frequently cry until it is replaced.

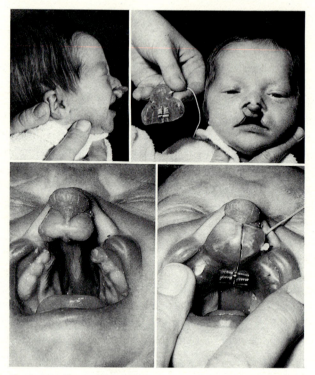

Fig. 1. Maxillary orthopedics. Split appliance, joined by reciprocating screw, used in child with complete bilateral cleft lip and palate. String is taped to face for security.

Maxillary orthopedics should be started as early as possible to take advantage of the rapid growth in the first few months of life. At this age, effective repositioning may be expected in 2–8 weeks, during which period the infant will have gained sufficiently to permit easier approximation of the lip segments. Once the lip is repaired, the reconstitution of the orbicularis oris muscle sphincter serves as a permanent splint for the newly positioned alveolar segments.

In some instances, the same effect may be achieved by recreating the orbicularis oris muscle sling of the lips with a relatively minor surgical procedure, commonly called the lip adhesion operation. The margins of the cleft are bared by the excision of an epithelial strip from each edge of the labial cleft and the raw surfaces are sutured together. Alternately, the epithelial covering of the cleft is fashioned into an anteriorly based (skin) flap on one side of the cleft and a posteriorly based (mucosa) flap on the other side. The

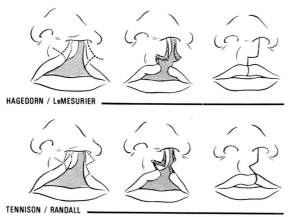

HAGEDORN / LeMESURIER

TENNISON / RANDALL   *Fig. 2.*

flaps are then sutured together. The definitive repair may be deferred until the child is deemed of an adequate age. This kind of management usually leads to a rather satisfactory overall result.

Surgery of Cleft Lip
Historical Background

Numerous procedures have been described for repair of congenital clefts of the lip. From the time of Celsus until well into the 19th century, the operation consisted of excision of the margins of the cleft and a crude approximation of the raw edges. At about 1830, DIEFFENBACH [7] introduced lateral undermining incisions to allow sliding of the flaps together with less tension. MIRAULT is generally credited with having been the first, in 1844, to bring a flap from the lateral segment across the lower margin of the cleft [14]. In the early 1930s, BLAIR and BROWN [6] applied MIRAULT's principle with better cosmetic results.

In 1880, JALAGUIER introduced a triangular flap from the lateral lip segment, which provided adequate lip height and a staggered scar [25]. HAGEDORN [12] devised a similar operation in 1884, but used a square flap instead. Through the years, many improvements and modifications in the various techniques have been made, largely through evaluation of postoperative results and self-criticism by the surgeons. Years later, LEMESURIER [13] popularized HAGEDORN's operation, while TENNISON [24] and RANDALL [2] reintroduced JALAGUIER's technique in simplified form (fig. 2).

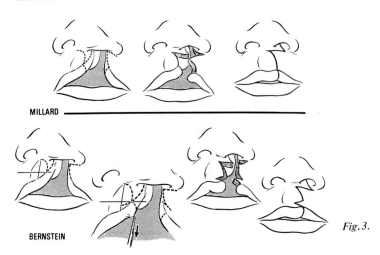

MILLARD

BERNSTEIN   *Fig. 3.*

One of the most outstanding contributions to improved cleft lip repair in recent years has been the rotation-advancement operation of MILLARD [15], although a precursor of it had already been published in 1901 by GIRALDÉ [25]. This is an excellent procedure for partial and narrow clefts. When combined with various refinements [18, 19], a most pleasing result may be expected. However, this operation requires artistic judgment, experience, and a high degree of skill. When applied to wider clefts, there is often a tendency to contraction of the main scar, so that a short lip may result. To help overcome difficulties that may be encountered in wide clefts, BERNSTEIN [4] modified MILLARD's rotation-advancement operation by incorporating a small triangular flap from the lateral segment into the bottom of the rotation flap (fig. 3).

Timing of Operation

Many surgeons feel that surgery should be delayed for at least 10 weeks following birth. By this time, the lip structures have increased in size, making the operative procedure easier and providing the surgeon with better tissues with which to work. There is actually little necessity for an early operation which can easily be delayed without seriously affecting the health of a newborn child. In general, this operation is postponed until the infant is steadily gaining weight and shows a normal blood count and an acceptable hemoglobin level. Ideally, it may be prudent to follow the minimum 'rule of ten' – at least 10 weeks of age, at least 10 lb. in weight, and at least 10 g of hemoglobin.

Operative Technique

The operation is performed under general anesthesia. A moist pack around the endotrachael tube is recommended to prevent aspiration of blood. It is preferable to schedule this operation as the first case in the morning, when the infant may not yet be very hungry, and to preclude the possibility of fatigue. Assuming an operative schedule that begins at 8 a.m. and the child on a 4-hourly feeding schedule, the last feeding is omitted.

The child is placed at the head of the table with its head slightly extended. The endotrachael tube is carefully taped in the middle of the lower lip to provide the least amount of lateral distortion. The eyes are taped shut and the exposed part of the face is cleansed with antiseptic soap. The operation is performed from the head of the table.

In this meticulous surgery, it is important to use instruments designed for fine, detailed work. Atraumatic technique with minimal manipulation of the tissues is important and wound margins should be handled with sharp skin hooks in order to avoid unnecessary trauma. Fine scalpels, small skin hooks, fine needle holders and small hemostats, a battery-powered ophthalmic cautery, and a fine pen comprise the basic armamentarium. Also necessary are fine-pointed calipers and a measuring rule. A weak local anesthetic solution with a vasoconstrictor is mandatory for hemostasis. A small suction tip and moist, cotton-tipped applicators are used to keep the small surgical field free of blood and to provide a clear field of vision for the surgeon.

The Unilateral Cleft Lip

This may perhaps be the first time that a detailed examination of the lip segments becomes possible. Prior to distorting the tissues with the local anesthetic solution, it is important to identify and mark with gentian violet solution the following landmarks (fig. 4): the bottom of Cupid's bow; the midpoint of attachment of the columella to the lip; the attachment of the alae to the lip; and the point at wich the vermilion of the cleft segment starts to become attenuated, which is usually identified by the sudden termination of the white ridge which normally exists at the vermilion-cutaneous (v-c) junction. These points are tattooed with a nonsiliconized hypodermic needle to prevent obliteration during the operation. It is particularly important to mark the exact vermilion border or the v-c ridge.

While it may be true that any of the operations in vogue nowadays will produce a satisfactory result in good hands, certain operations have advantages over others. Yet, the surgeon is encouraged to acquaint himself with

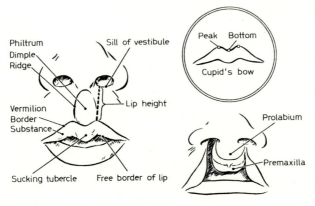

Fig.4.

the various operative procedures available, so as to avoid creating the circumstance where the lip is made to fit the procedure and not vice versa. Furthermore, familiarity with the various procedures, hopefully, may lead to the development of improved modifications. Since there are several different operative techniques available, and the choice is dependent upon the preference of the surgeon and the type of case under consideration, only the principles of the operative procedure will be discussed.

Ideally, the operation should be designed to meet the following criteria: (1) accurate approximation of skin, muscle, and mucosa; (2) an inconspicuous scar; (3) symmetric lip length; (4) creation of a symmetric Cupid's bow; (5) creation of a philtrum dimple; (6) slight eversion, or pouting, of the lip; (7) symmetric nostrils; (8) a symmetric columella; (9) creation of a labial sulcus, and (10) easy adaptability of the procedure to various clefts.

It is essentail that the tissues be cut sharply, with clear incisive strokes of the knife held at right angles to the skin's surface. The skin having been incised squarely, the knife may be slanted toward the cleft so as to preserve as much muscle and mucosa as possible. Bleeding points may be grasped with very small hemostats, which are left on for several minutes. In most instances, this will suffice to control hemorrhage, obviating the use of buried sutures. Nevertheless, a battery-powered ophthalmic cautery may be desirable to control specific bleeding points. When ligation of the coronary vessels is needed, 5–0 chromic catgut may be used.

In preparing the flaps, it is often necessary to release the lip segments from their attachments to the underlying bone. This may not be required on the uncleft side in every case, however. When needed, only a minimal amount of undermining should be done, just sufficient to permit approximation of the flaps. On the cleft side, care should be taken to avoid the infraorbital nerve which emerges at a relatively lower level in infants. In very wide clefts, the ala on the cleft side may have to be detached completely from the maxilla in order to facilitate approximation of the lip segments.

In the presence of an underlying cleft of the alveolar process, this may be closed simultaneously with repair of the lip. The autor favors the technique described by Skoog [22], which creates a partial sleeve from the mucoperiosteum that lines the alveolar cleft. The anterior defect of this 'sleeve' is closed by creating a medially based flap of periosteum from the anterior part of the maxilla and rotating it through 180° to bridge the alveolar gap. The space between this maxillary periosteum and the mucoperiosteum that had been sutured within the cleft may be filled with small pieces of Gelfoam or with blood clot.

Fine chromic catgut sutures are used for the muscle layer and 6–0 nylon for the skin closure. It is customary to close the mucosal surface with fine chromic sutures. Care must be taken with placement of the sutures, and that they not be tied too tightly. The skin sutures should suffice merely to approximate the skin edges.

Dissection of the asymmetric tip cartilage of the nose on the cleft side, simultaneously with lip repair, should only be undertaken by experienced surgeons; however, a certain degree of repositioning is being done more and more frequently. When the tip cartilage has been freed, a through-and-through mattress suture, tied over bolsters, is useful for coapting the tissue layers in the new position.

A lip dressing is not necessary, but the line of suture may be covered with bland ophthalmic ointment. Before removing the endotracheal tube, the pharynx is suctioned for any residual blood clots. This is repeated on removal of the tube. The child is then taken to the recovery room and is kept in a croupette for 24 h. The infant's arms are restrained by splinting at the elbows, and he is prevented from turning onto his face by pinning his arms to the bedsheets in the supine position.

Postoperative feeding is given by some form of syringe as described above. The suture line is cleansed after meals with hydrogen peroxide and the ophthalmic ointment is reapplied. Intermittent skin sutures may be removed on the third or fourth postoperative day, retaining the sutures at key points until the fifth day. The sutures should be removed with meticulous care. The head needs to be restrained, either by a firm pair of hands or by means of a wide adhesive bandage which straps the head to the table. The child may need to be sedated. On the other hand, it may work equally well if removal of the sutures is timed just before a meal, when the child is hungry. A small wad of qauze, soaked in sugar water and placed in the mouth on the side away from the cleft, will often suffice to distract the hungry infant. After the sutures have been removed, the wound edges may be supported with adhesive strips for several days.

The Bilateral Cleft Lip

Best results are usually obtained in these patients by repairing one side at a time, with an interval of about 3 months. Rarely, such management may not be feasible because of a protrusive premaxilla. In planning the treatment, the following principles are recommended:

(1) Maxillary orthopedics should be instituted to improve the position of the three components of the alveolar arch. In bilateral cleft lip and palate, the object of the orthopedic appliance is to hold the premaxilla back while opening the maxillary segments to accommodate the premaxilla. If the maxillary segments are not collapsed behind the premaxilla, then the appliance serves to promote forward movement of these segments to meet with the premaxilla, which is being held back meanwhile.

(2) The prolabium should be used to form the full vertical length of the middle of the lip, assuming it to be the total contribution to the philtrum. At a cursory glance, the prolabium appears to be entirely inadequate for reconstituting the full vertical height of the middle of the lip. Having a narrow attachment, the natural elasticity of the skin causes it to contract toward the columella. Moreover, because it has little or no muscle, it is thinner than the lateral lip segments.

(3) The curved v-c border at the bottom of the philtrum should provide the central convexity of Cupid's bow.

(4) The midportion of the vermilion should be built up with vermilion-muscle flaps taken from the lateral lip segments.

(5) Bilateral lip repair should take into consideration the almost inevitable need for revision at a later date. For this reason, as much tissue as possible should be preserved, to have it available for future revision.

As with the unilateral cleft, the simplest form of bilateral cleft lip is when the defect is only partial. As the degree of deformity increases, it is usually compounded by the increased involvement of the underlying bony framework and is further aggravated yet when the premaxilla is protrusive.

In partial and in complete clefts, in which the premaxilla is not too prominent, the rotation-advancement method may be applied in two separate operations [17]. There are distinct cosmetic advantages of this operation (fig. 5, III). In moderately protrusive cases, the straight line repair of Veau may be used in one stage, but preferably should be in two, since the latter gives better cosmetic results (fig. 5, I).

A certain amount of spontaneous recession of the premaxilla may be expected postoperatively as a result of changes in the muscular forces acting on the palatal segments. Thus, in markedly protrusive cases, a straight line coaptation of the lip segments may be attempted, its main object being to reconstitute the orbicularis oris muscle sling in order to achieve some improved repositioning of the segments.

The SCHULTZ [21] method may be used for closing bilateral clefts of the lip with a protrusive premaxilla where the lip segments may have to be approximated under some degree of tension (fig. 5, II). When it is well indicated, this is a satisfactory method of achieving both immediate bilateral lip closure and fairly rapid repositioning of the premaxilla, provided the maxillary segments are sufficiently apart to receive it. This operation also provides a labial sulcus over the premaxilla.

In very rare cases, there may be an indication for surgical recession of the premaxilla, or for its resection. This should only be done when it is quite impossible to effect lip closure. Because of the danger of interference with midfacial growth when such a procedure is performed so early in life, great caution should be exercised in selecting patients for such an operation.

Surgery of Cleft Palate

The development of the surgical closure of the cleft palate is a long and fascinating story and its details are beyond the scope of this chapter. It was VON LANGENBECK [8] who introduced the technique of creating mucoperiosteal flaps through lateral incisions in 1861 which in essence were two bipedicled flaps freed from their underlying bone and sutured in the midline (fig. 6, I). Because many of these patients exhibited postoperative shortening of the palate, in 1895 SMITH [23] of Nashua, New Hampshire, devised a method of retropositioning the soft palate by means of four flaps (fig. 6, III), while GANZER [10] introduced the three-flap retrodisplacement operation in 1920 (fig. 6, II). Modern day palatal surgery embodies the basic principles as introduced by VAN LANGENBECK, SMITH, and GANZER

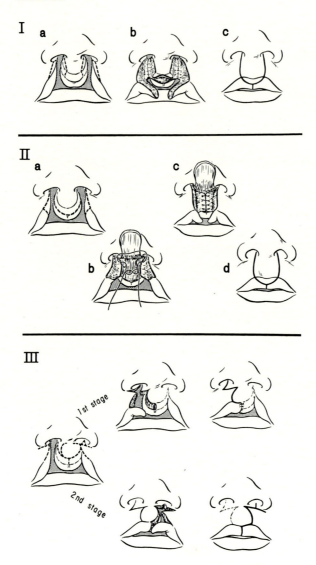

Fig.5. Operations for bilateral cleft lip: (I) Veau, done in one or two stages; (II) Schultz, done in one stage; (III) Millard, done in two stages.

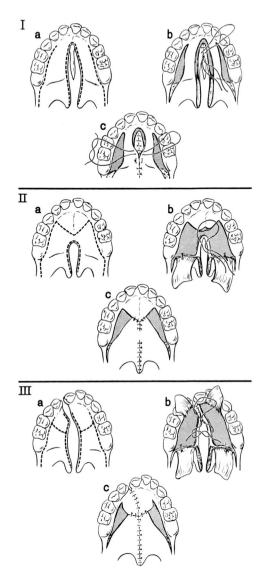

Fig.6. Operations for cleft palate: (I) modified Langenbeck repair in cleft of secondary palate; (II) the three-flap pushback operation; (III) the four-flap pushback repair. In each case, *a* shows the incisions, *b* elevated flaps and suture of nasal mucosa, and *c* the final suturing.

and numerous other contributors [8], each of whom added specific refinements.

The ideal cleft palate operation should aim at the following requirements: (1) closure of the cleft of the palate in one operation; (2) elongating the palate, or at least preventing its postoperative shortening; (3) preservation of normal function of the velum; (4) achieving adequate velopharyngeal competence; (5) normal speech production; (6) normally functioning auditory tubes; (7) a normal masticatory apparatus without malocclusion; (8) minimal interference with underlying bone growth; (9) the avoidance of facial deformity, and (10) no interference with normal nasal physiology.

Timing the Operation

In determining the optimal timing of the cleft palate operation, the surgeon needs to take into consideration the effect that such timing may have on speech on the one hand, and on underlying bone growth on the other hand. Several well-documented studies have shown that if repair is carried out after the deciduous dentition has erupted, the amount of retardation of postoperative facial growth is minimal. On the other hand, it is generally agreed that better speech patterns result if the operation is done at an early age. Thus, in order to satisfy both requirements, it is quite reasonable to schedule the operation sometime between the ages of 24 and 36 months [3].

Operative Technique

As with the lip operation, the child should be in good health, with an adequate hemoglobin level and normal blood count. The operation is done in the Rose position with endotracheal anesthesia. Moist gauze is loosely packed around the tube in the hypopharynx to prevent aspiration of blood. Various mouth gags are available which have been specifically designed for this operation.

The operative technique should incorporate the following principles:

Hemostasis. This is greatly aided by infiltrating the operative field with a weak local anesthetic solution containing a vasoconstrictor. Bleeding points are controlled with weak electrocautery.

Conservation of tissue. Meticulous care is necessary in the handling of the tissues, and crushing must be avoided at all times. Fine skin hooks should be used instead of forceps. No tissue is ever discarded. Adequate mobilization of flaps is necessary and strangulation of tissues by tight sutures is to be avoided, to prevent tension and necrosis along the line of repair.

Mucosal coverage of cleft. To minimize postoperative contraction and to effect a stronger repair line, it is necessary to cover the cleft with mucosa on the nasal as well as the oral surfaces. The nasal flap may be augmented at the expense of the oral mucosa by placing the oral incision 2–3 mm lateral to the cleft (fig. 6). The nasal mucosa is then freed from its bony attachement to facilitate its medial advancement.

In unilateral clefts, the nasal mucoperiosteum on the cleft side must be sutured to the mucosal flap covering the vomer. In bilateral complete clefts, and in clefts of the secondary palate, the vomerine flaps should be so utilized whenever possible.

Retrodisplacement of velum. Closure of the cleft in a simple approximation of the mucoperiosteal flaps will lead to shortening of the palate on healing. To avoid this, and to compensate for the congenital underdevelopment of the tissues, the soft palate musculature is freed from the posterior edge of the bony palate; however, the nasal mucosa is kept intact at this level. This facilitates both retrodisplacement and medial advancement of the velum. The new position is maintained by the V-Y three- or four-flap technique (fig. 6, II and III).

In patients with wide clefts, or with very short palates, this maneuver will be greatly aided by freeing or cutting the greater palatine neurovascular bundle.

At the conclusion of the operation, the surgical field should be completely dry. The pharynx is aspirated of any blood clots, and this is repeated after the endotracheal tube is removed. The patient is taken to the recovery room where he is placed in a croupette in which he is kept for 24 h. The patient is kept on a liquid diet by cup feeding until healing has taken place, some 3 weeks later. Arm restraints are applied to prevent the child from tugging on the ends of the sutures or from placing a potentially harmful object in the mouth. The patient is usually discharged from hospital a week after the operation.

Further Management
Speech therapy. Speech therapy is generally avoided for approximately 1 year after the repair of the cleft palate, since it takes about that long for the scar tissue to settle. With speech therapy, and in a well-controlled

environment, approximately 60–80 % of repaired cleft palate patients should achieve satisfactory speech production with good velopharyngeal competence. In those patients in whom velopharyngeal competence is not achieved, in spite of intensive and prolonged speech therapy, a surgical procedure or a dental obturator may be indicated to diminish the velopharyngeal aperture.

Otitis media. The incidence of nonsuppurative otitis media is extremely high in cleft palate children. That this is due to malfunction of the auditory tube is generally accepted. However, all of the reasons for the malfunction are not clearly understood, because satisfactory repair of the palate does not automatically restore normal function to the tube.

Excluding instances of suppurative otitis media, attention is first given to the ears of cleft palate babies at about 10–12 months of age, when the babble pattern of speech begins. If nonsuppurative otitis media is encountered, myringotomies are performed and ventilating tubes are inserted through them. Thereafter, the ears are examined at intervals of about 6 months. The procedure of myringotomies and the insertion of tubes is repeated periodically as indicated; however, the need for this diminishes with growth and usually peters out toward the end of the first decade of life.

Adenoidectomy is deemed inadvisable in these patients because of the immediate deterioration of speech, unless a pharyngeal flap operation is anticipated. Whereas a child with good speech usually adjusts quite easily to the infinitesimally slow physiologic regression of the adenoid pad, it is too much to expect him to compensate for the sudden removal of this tissue. Accordingly, in the interest of maintaining existing good speech in cleft palate children, treatment of otitis media should not include adenoidectomy.

Orthodontics. A rather high proportion of complete clefts of the palate will eventually require various degrees of orthodontic management. This is usually initiated at the time of the mixed dentition, and such patients should be handled by orthodontists who are well acquainted with the problems of the cleft palate patient.

Secondary Problems in Maxillofacial Clefts

Velopharyngeal incompetence. This condition exists in 20–40 % of patients operated for clefts of the palate. It is also frequently found in those with submucous clefts. Depending on the amount of incompetence, as determined by physical examination, speech results, oral breath pressure ratios, and lateral pharyngeal radiographs, the modality of treatment may be determined [2]. This may consist of a dental obturator designed to lift the velum to a higher plane in order to assist its articulation with the posterior pharyngeal wall; however, its value is rather limited.

Surgical correction consists either of the creation of a pharyngeal pad, or a pharyngeal flap, or the injection of Teflon paste into the posterior pharyngeal wall. The pharyngeal flap operation, or velopharyngoplasty, is usually undertaken at about 6 or 7 years of age, after an adequate period of intensive speech therapy, and after a full evaluation of the velopharyngeal incompetence. This operation may also be indicated in cases of postoperative breakdown of a repaired cleft of the velum. In younger children, and in those of slight built, it may very occasionally become imperative to do a tracheostomy postoperatively because of edema in the hypopharynx. Once the decision for a pharyngeal flap procedure has been made, it is prudent to remove enlarged adenoids about 6–12 weeks prior to the date of the velopharyngoplasty.

The operation is done in the Rose position with endotracheal intubation. A weak anesthetic-vasoconstrictor solution is infiltrated into the posterior pharyngeal wall and the free edge of the palate. A superiorly based flap is outlined to include most of the width of the posterior pharyngeal wall extending from the plane of the velum almost to the level of the tip of the epiglottis. The mucomuscular flap is freed from the underlying alar fascia with blunt scissors dissection.

The free edge of the velum is split horizontally between the oral and nasal surfaces, thus creating the recipient bed (fig. 7). This extends laterally about halfway down the posterior pillar of the fauces, to leave adequate lateral portals for nasal respiration.

A modification of this operation was recently reported by BERNSTEIN [5]. To prevent the pharyngeal flap from excessively tubing itself, thus becoming narrow and less effectual in some cases, a secondary flap is created to partially cover the raw surfaces of the larger flap. The lesser flap is fashioned from the posterior edge of the nasal surface of the soft palate. This necessitates anchoring the pharyngeal flap to the velum along a more advanced recipient bed. The author is of the opinion that this makes the flap more efficient.

A certain degree of temporary neck rigidity is not an unusual postoperative phenomenon. Swallowing is rather difficult, and this must be

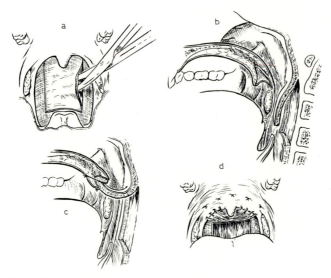

Fig.7. Steps in the pharyngeal flap operation.

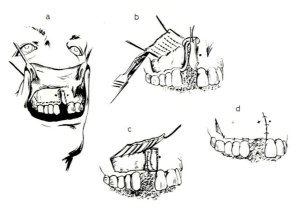

Fig.8. Method of closing nasolabial fistula. *a* Outline of flaps. *b* Periosteum incised in parallel grid to allow larger flap to stretch.

vigoriously encouraged. The patient is discharged from hospital after about a week and is kept on a liquid diet for about 3 weeks. Because of edema, the lateral airway portals may be closed for several weeks postoperatively. Improvement in speech is frequently apparent soon after the operation, but no therapy is given for about 3–6 months.

Fistulas. Apart from velopharyngeal incompetence, a wide nasolabial fistula may also be responsible for air escape during speech, in addition to spillage of food into the nose. In such instances this may have to be closed using local mucoperiosteal flaps (fig. 8). In some institutions, this procedure is combined with the insertion of a bone graft.

Oronasal fistulas usually result from partial breakdown of the repair line, except for the very narrow fistulas in the region of the alveolar process. Symptomatic fistulas may be closed surgically, or they may be covered with a dental appliance.

Esthetic problems. In addition to the treatment of velopharyngeal incompetence, most secondary operations are concerned with problems of esthetics. Of these, the nose holds a very high priority. In line with the frequent need for septal reconstruction in unilateral clefts of the palate, the external nose in these cases is almost always asymmetric.

If the bony pyramid requires reduction, it is best to delay doing the rhinoplasty until the patient is well into the teens. However, a soft tissue rhinoplastic procedure may be undertaken earlier. The common deformity specifically consists of a distorted and often underdeveloped tip cartilage on the cleft side, the cartilage being asymmetrically placed in relation to its opposite fellow. Often, there is also distortion of the nostril, especially manifested by a weblike fold across the apex of the naris and a caudal displacement of the rim.

The bilateral cleft nose, on the other hand, invariably presents with a short columella and wide, flaring nares. A very satisfactory method of elongating the columella is that described by MILLARD [16], but this should be done only when the quadrilateral septal cartilage begins to exert pull on the short columella (fig. 9).

Other frequently performed procedures on cleft lip children are concerned with revision of the lip scar, realignment of the v-c border (fig. 10), and augmentation of the vermilion substance of the lip [1]. If the lip is short on the cleft side, and when a 'whistling' deformity is present, the scar revision should include a lengthening procedure (fig. 11). Because some of the older lip operations did not preserve the Cupid's bow, it may be reconstructed in such cases by advancing the v-c border into a symmetric pattern of the bow (fig. 12). Deficiencies at the free border of the vermilion may be augmented by rolling out the mucous membrane of the inside of the lip (fig. 13).

The labial sulcus in bilateral clefts is invariably nonexistent, or may be very shallow, as a result of attachment of the prolabium to the premaxilla.

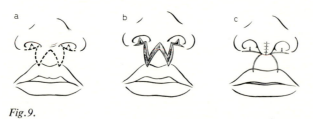

Fig. 9.

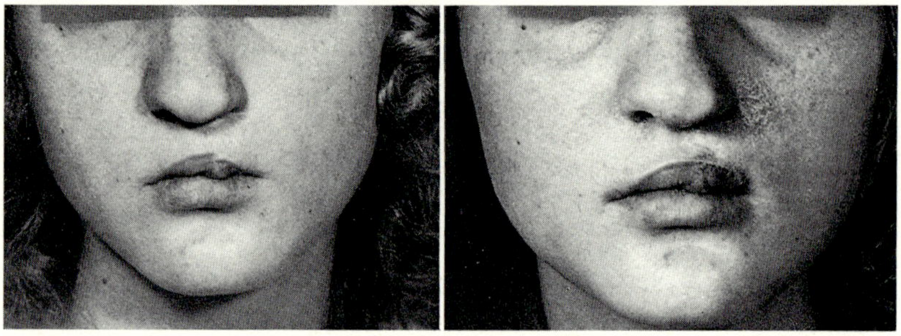

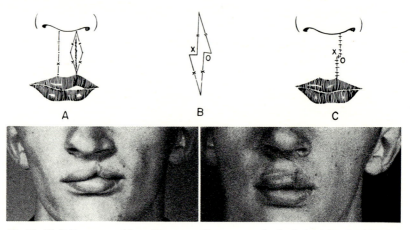

Fig. 10. Correction of malposed vermilion by means of Z-plasty.

Fig. 11. Cleft lip scar revision. Diagrams illustrate method of obtaining lengthening and a staggered scar to eliminate the 'whistling deformity' and to preclude further contraction.

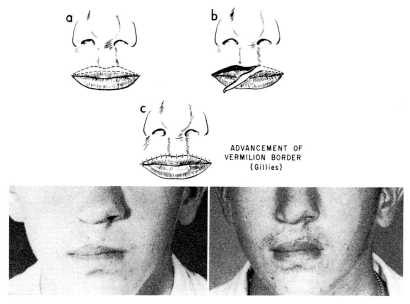

ADVANCEMENT OF
VERMILION BORDER
(Gillies)

Fig. 12.

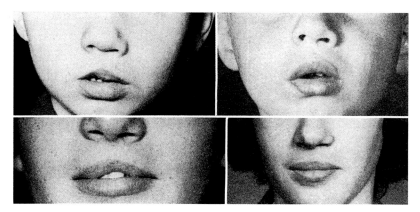

Fig. 13. Vermilion augmentation. Top, unilateral; bottom, central.

This ties the lip down, necessitating the creation of a sulcus to allow the lip to move freely. The sulcus may be lined with a split thickness skin graft or with dermis; alternately, the newly created space may be maintained by means of a dental obturator until epithelialization has taken place in about 14 days.

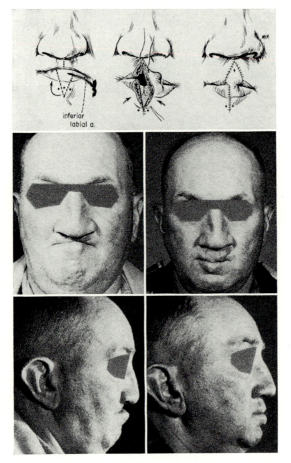

inferior
labial a.

Fig. 14. The Abbe procedure. The illustration shows the steps of the first stage. The photographs on the right show the final result some years later (nothing else had been done at this stage).

In some bilateral clefts, the upper lip may be short and tight, either as a result of underdeveloped tissues, or because of aggresive surgery; or for both reasons. Consequently, there may be marked discrepancy between the two lips. The condition may be greatly improved by augmenting the upper midportion of the lip with a triangular full-thickness flap from the lower lip – the Abbe operation (fig. 14).

References

1 BERNSTEIN, L.: Secondary reconstructive procedures for cleft lip and nose. Trans. Am. Acad. Ophthal. Oto-la. *71:* 71–80 (1967).

2 BERNSTEIN, L.: Treatment of velopharyngeal incompetence. Archs Otolar. *85:* 67–74 (1967).

3 BERNSTEIN, L.: The effect of timing of cleft palate operations on subsequent growth of the maxilla. Laryngoscope *78:* 1510–1565 (1968).

4 BERNSTEIN, L.: Modified operation for wide unilateral cleft lips. Archs Otolar. *91:* 11–18 (1970).

5 BERNSTEIN, L.: A modified pharyngeal flap operation. Trans. Am. Acad. Ophthal. Oto-lar. *80:* 514–518 (1975).

6 BLAIR, V. P. and BROWN, J. B.: Mirault operation for single harelip. Surgery Gynec. Obstet. *51:* 81–98 (1930).

7 DIEFFENBACH, J. F.: Die Operative Chirurgie (Brockhaus, Leipzig 1845).

8 DORRANCE, G. M.: The operative story of cleft palate (Saunders, Philadelphia 1933).

9 DOUGLAS, B.: The treatment of micrognathia associated with obstruction by a plastic procedure. Plastic reconstr. Surg. *1:* 300–308 (1946).

10 GANZER, H.: Wolfsrachenplastik mit Ausnutzung des gesamten Schleimhaut-materials zur Vermeidung der Verkürzung des Gaumensegels. Berl. klin. Wschr. *57:* 619 (1920).

11 GORLIN, R. J. and PINDBORG, J. J.: Syndromes of the head and neck (Blakiston Division, McGraw-Hill, New York 1964).

12 HAGEDORN, W.: Über eine Modifikation der Hasenschartenoperation. Zentbl. Chir. *11:* 756–758 (1884).

13 LEMESURIER, A. B.: A method of cutting and suturing the lip in the treatment of complete unilateral clefts. Plastic reconstr. Surg. *4:* 1–12 (1949).

14 MCDOWELL, F.: Late results in cleft lip repairs. Plastic reconstr. Surg. *38:* 444–476 (1966).

15 MILLARD, D. R.: A primary camouflage in the unilateral hare lip; in SKOOG Trans. 1st Int. Congr. Plastic Surgeons, p. 160 (Williams & Wilkins, Baltimore 1957).

16 MILLARD, D. R.: Columella lengthening by the forked flap. Plastic reconstr. Surg. *22:* 454–457 (1958).

17 MILLARD, D. R.: Adaptation of rotation-advancement principle in bilateral cleft lip. Trans. Int. Soc. Plast. Surg., vol. 2, p. 50 (1960).

18 MILLARD, D. R.: Refinements in rotation-advancement cleft lip technique. Plastic reconstr. Surg. *33:* 26–38 (1964).

19 MILLARD, D. R.: Extensions of the rotation-advancement principle for wide uni-lateral cleft lips. Plastic reconstr. Surg. *42:* 535–544 (1968).

20 RANDALL, P.: A triangular flap operation for the primary repair of unilateral clefts of the lip. Plastic reconstr. Surg. *23:* 331–347 (1959).

21 SCHULTZ, L. W.: Bilateral cleft lips. Plastic reconstr. Surg. *1:* 338–343 (1946).

22 SKOOG, T.: The use of periosteum and surgical for bone restoration in congenital clefts of the maxilla. Scand. J. Plast. reconstr. Surg. *1:* 113–130 (1967).

23 SMITH, H. L.: Cleft palate. Boston med. Surg. J. *132:* 478 (1895).

24   TENNISON, C.W.: The repair of the unilateral cleft lip by the stencil method. Plastic
      reconstr.Surg. *9:* 115–120 (1952).
25   THOMPSON, J.E.: An artistic and mathematically accurate method of repairing the
      defect in cases of hare-lip. Surgery Gynec.Obstet. *14:* 498–505 (1912).
26   WASHIO, H.: History of cleft lip surgery; in STARK Cleft palate (Holt Medical Divi-
      sion, Harper & Row, New York 1968).

L.BERNSTEIN, MD, DDS, Professor and Chairman, Department of Otorhinolaryngology,
University of California, Davis 4301 X Street, Suite 208, *Sacramento, CA 95817* (USA)

Adv. Oto-Rhino-Laryng., vol. 23, pp. 155–168 (Karger, Basel 1978)

Maxillofacial Injury

BYRON J. BAILEY and VINCENT H. CARUSO

Department of Otolaryngology, The University of Texas Medical Branch, Galveston, Tex.

Introduction

The broad field of trauma is relevant to any review of pediatric otolaryngology. *Accident Facts* [8], published by the National Safety Council, states that accidents are the leading cause of death for American children between the ages of 1 and 14 years. In fact, accidents are responsible for 46 % of the deaths in this group, and those involving motor vehicles are the largest group within this category.

The morbidity, functional deficits, and deformities associated with facial trauma are also significant factors in this age group. Many authors have emphasized the emotional anguish and economic costs to society caused by trauma in our modern culture, but despite these efforts, the field remains relatively fragmented or neglected in many communities.

The purpose of this chapter is to emphasize recent advances in the management of maxillofacial injuries in children. We also attempt to clarify some of the controversial issues in this area and to emphasize the importance of the 'team concept' in hospital management.

Otologic Injuries

Impedance audiometry is of great help in diagnosing otologic injuries in children. The tympanogram aids in determining the status of the ossicular chain when the tympanic membrane is intact. Ossicular discontinuity, which may result from a fall or blow to the head, may be overlooked in children who are too young for precise audiometry. In these patients, tympanometry provides an indication of the status of the ossicular chain, and an ossicular discontinuity may be diagnosed. A conductive hearing loss may also be suspected on stapedius reflex testing. In addition, electrocochleography, in combination with stapedius reflex testing and other techniques of audiometry, may provide an indication of the overall hearing in infants and young children. The audiogram, pneumootoscopy, impedance audiometry, and electrocochleography are all available for diagnostic purposes. The vestibular test battery is helpful in diagnosing labyrinthine and eighth nerve injuries resulting from temporal bone fractures in children. The torsion swing test will indicate the presence of a recent ablative lesion of the vestibular labyrinth and show central compensation. This last test is easy to perform in infants and children when they are held in an adult's lap in the chair.

Children presenting with a history of head trauma, progressive hearing loss, tinnitus, and vertigo should be evaluated for the possibility of oval or round window rupture with perilymph fistula. This is particularly true if a positive fistula test is elicited or if fluid is noted behind the tympanic membrane on otoscopy. When the presence of a fistula is suspected, an exploratory tympanotomy should be performed. The round and oval windows should be observed using the 25 power objective of the microscope for a minimum of 5 min. The physician looks for the accumulation of clear fluid in an otherwise dry area in the round and oval windows.

Repair of a fistula will prevent subsequent episodes of meningitis as well as further hearing loss. A fistula repair is accomplished by denuding the mucosa overlying the stapes footplate or around the round window niche and placing a lobular fat graft into the fistula site. The patient is maintained in a head-elevated position for 12 h to lower the cerebrospinal fluid and perilymph pressure. Hearing may improve and vertigo disappear dramatically following this repair.

Soft Tissue Injuries

Patients are now more knowledgeable about plastic reconstructive surgery and are demanding optimal results following repair of traumatic injuries. Facial lacerations must be handled appropriately in the emergency room, using plastic soft tissue techniques to obtain the ideal cosmetic results. Among the new instruments that are helpful in these cases is the bipolar forceps cautery, which allows the surgeon to coagulate small vessels very precisely without causing burns to adjacent tissue. This decreases the amount of necrotic tissue within the wound and thereby decreases the opportunity for infection. In the initial repair of lacerations that do not follow relaxed skin tension lines, the wound may be closed primarily because of the difficulty in accurately determining the extent of the devitalized tissue, the beveled nature of the borders of the laceration, and the likelihood of hematoma and infection complicating the wound trauma. In addition, the parents might look unfavorably upon the results unless they have seen the scars that would have resulted from the injury had less sophisticated techniques been used. The surgeon should be familiar with all of the available techniques, as described in depth in the recent text by BORGES [1]. The use of Davis and Geck 6–0 mild chromic catgut® for skin closure with taping is described by WEBSTER *et al.* [10]. This gives a fine cosmetic result and allows quick, atraumatic suture removal in a young child, since the suture comes out when the tape comes off.

Nasal Injuries

The nose is relatively smaller and has less tip projection in the child than in the adult. In the newborn, the length of the nasal bones nearly equals their width, whereas in the adult the length is three times the width. Therefore, nasal injuries in the infant and young child are less common than in the older child and adult. Nasal fracture reduction is undergoing some modification, since rhinoplastic surgeons are now inclined to perform open reductions under direct visualization. This reduction may be performed through intercartilaginous incisions that allow precise reduction of the fracture with removal of periosteum and soft tissue from between bony fragments. Using this technique, the nasal bones are less likely to drift back to their prereduction state as healing takes place, and there is no additional interference with the growth centers that has not already occurred as a result of the trauma.

Fractures of the Maxilla

The most widely accepted system for classification of maxillary fractures is that described by LE FORT [7] in 1900. In addition to the classical horizontal fractures, there are a variety of incomplete maxillary fractures that involve the alveolar ridge, the anterior or lateral maxillary wall, and the inferior orbital rim.

The classical Le Fort horizontal fractures are seen infrequently in children under the age of 8 years because of the thick, strong maxillary wall that is present before the antrum has developed fully. As facial development progresses and the eruption of permanent dentition is completed, the same fracture pattern as seen in adults begin to occur.

Diagnostic features of these maxillary fractures include palpable bony deformity, moderate to severe soft tissue swelling, epistaxis, cerebrospinal fluid rhinorrhea, anesthesia of the cheek in the distribution of the infraorbital nerve, nasal obstruction, anosmia, epiphora, diplopia, 'dish face' deformity, and malocclusion in any combination.

Careful palpation of the maxilla may disclose a step-off deformity of the infraorbital rim or subcutaneous emphysema of the facial skin. Presence of the fracture may be confirmed by the detection of maxillary mobility when the central incisor is grasped firmly and rocked gently.

Roentgenographic examination, especially the use of polytomography, is extremely useful in determining the exact location of the fracture lines.

Treatment is individualized, and the general principle of employing the smallest surgical procedure likely to produce a satisfactory result should be followed. The major importance of midfacial fractures lies in the degree to which they result in one of the following: (1) ocular dysfunction; (2) malocclusion, and (3) deformity of facial contour.

Le Fort I Fractures

Figure 1A shows the typical location of a Le Fort I fracture. Note that in the child with unerupted dentition, it is not uncommon for the fracture line to extend across the area of an unerupted tooth. The parents should be given a clear explanation about the possibility of abnormal or delayed tooth eruption. The point should be made to the parents that this abnormality is the result of the trauma sustained in the injury, not the result of the subsequent surgical management. The immediate goal of treatment is to obtain immobilization of the fracture in good anatomic position and with optimal occlusion. Consultation and collaboration with a dentist is an important part of the team management for this injury.

In figure 1B, the treatment for a typical fracture of this type is illustrated. Note that there are three circumferential wires supporting the mandibular arch bar and four supporting the maxillary arch bar. Individual wire ligatures are also placed around each tooth and are even more necessary in the pediatric patient than in the adult because of the ease with which deciduous teeth can be avulsed. Although not shown in figure 1B, individual

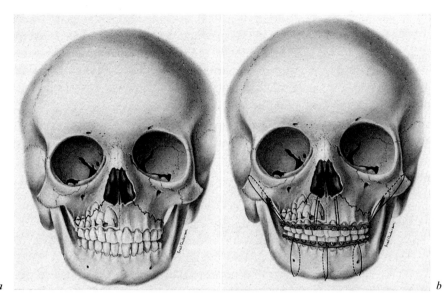

a   b

Fig. 1. A Le Fort I fracture of the maxilla. Note the involvement of tooth buds.
B Repair of fracture employing arch bars and elastic bands. Note the circumferential
wiring around the mandible and the supporting suspension wires around the zygomatic
arches and from the pyriform apertures.

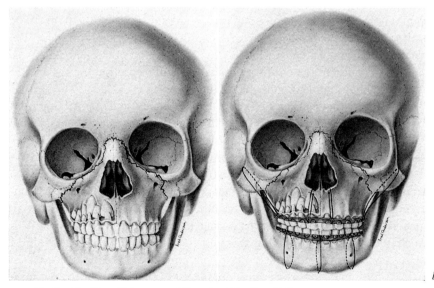

a   b

Fig. 2. A Le Fort II fracture. *B* Repair of Le Fort II fracture.

dental ligatures are applied to all available teeth, except the central and lateral incisors. Four to six dental elastic bands ($\frac{3}{8}$ inch) are placed between the upper and lower arch bars on each side. This arrangement allows the teeth to be held in good approximation and in occlusion during the period of healing. The appliance is left in place for approximately 4 weeks, a time sufficient to assure healing in the pediatric patient.

Le Fort II Fractures

The Le Fort II or pyramidal fracture is illustrated in figure 2 A. In most instances, this fracture is caused by a high velocity impact across the dorsum of the nose and results in a separation through the nasal bones and passing inferiorly to the zygomatic complex. Ocular complications are uncommon, but the physician needs to be aware that they may accompany this fracture. Consultation and collaboration with an ophthalmologist is important in these cases as well as in cases of Le Fort III fractures.

The usual management for a Le Fort II fracture is illustrated in figure 2 B. This technique of repair employs the same principles as the Le Fort I fracture, and the comments that have been made above also pertain to the Le Fort II fracture.

Le Fort III Fractures

This fracture is essentially a separation of the facial bones from the cranium (fig. 3 A). The fracture line usually extends through the floor of the orbit, and ocular complications of some degree are usually present. The fracture lines may extend to involve the frontal and ethmoidal sinuses as well as the region of the cribriform plate. Careful inspection for evidence of a cerebrospinal fluid leak must be routine.

The forces that cause a Le Fort III fracture are usually quite large, and the physician must have a high index of suspicion for a possible basal skull fracture and associated neurological complications. Appropriate neurosurgical consultation is indicated, since this injury may be life-threatening.

The management of the Le Fort III fracture is shown in figure 3 B. In addition to the application of dental arch bars and reinforcing circumferential mandibular supporting wires, the best reduction is obtained by an open reduction and interosseous wiring at the upper fracture line. This usually occurs at the zygomatic-frontal suture line, and the point of direct interosseous wiring is also the point of placement for the lateral suspension wires. Additional supporting wires are placed in the region of the pyriform aperture and extend down to the region of the maxillary incisors. Immobili-

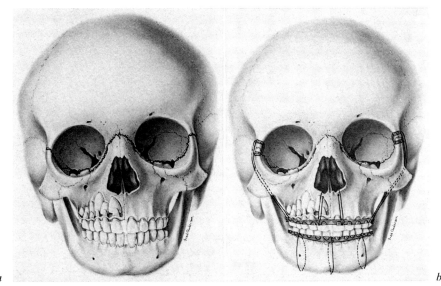

Fig.3. A Le Fort III fracture (craniofacial separation). *B* Repair of Le Fort III fracture.

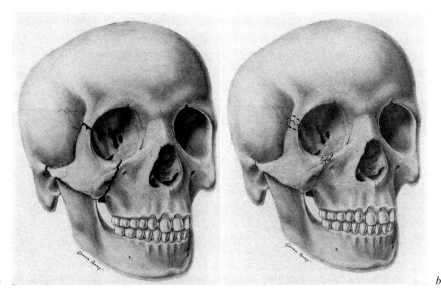

Fig.4. A Fracture of the zygoma. *B* Repair of zygomatic fracture at two points, using direct interosseous wiring.

zation in occlusion should be maintained for 4–5 weeks, depending upon the severity of the injury. External fixation appliances are seldom necessary.

Fractures of the Zygoma

Zygomatic or tripod fractures are usually the result of trauma sustained from an automobile or sports accident or from a physical assault. These injuries may be associated with ocular dysfunction, which is usually not serious unless there has been trauma directly to the orbit. Because of the thickness of the bone in this area prior to full development of the maxillary sinus, these fractures are uncommon in younger children. Subconjunctival hemorrhage is a common finding with these injuries.

A typical zygomatic fracture is shown in figure 4A. The fracture line is usually near the zygomatic-frontal and the zygomatic-maxillary suture lines. There is a fracture across the zygomatic arch, usually at a weak point in the zygomatic extension of the temporal bone. Inadequate management of this fracture will often result in the inferior displacement of the lateral canthus of the eye as well as a significant deformity of the prominence and contour of the cheek on the involved side.

When treating the pediatric patient with this fracture, the Caldwell-Luc approach should be avoided because of the possibility of injury to unerupted tooth buds. As shown in figure 4B, the two-point fixation at the lateral orbital rim and the inferior orbital rim will facilitate healing of the zygomatic fragment in good anatomic position. These two sites for direct interossesous wiring are accessible through small incisions in skin creases in the temporal and infraorbital regions.

Orbital Floor 'Blow-Out' Fractures

The classical orbital floor 'blow-out' fracture and its treatment were described initially by CONVERSE and SMITH [3]. This fracture occurs when a large force is applied directly over the orbit from anteriorly. Such a blow may create a comminuted fracture of the weakest portion of the orbital cavity, the floor of the orbit. This fracture may result in herniation of orbital fat into the maxillary antrum, with or without entrapment of the inferior rectus muscle.

The injury may be associated with enophthalmos, diplopia, or serious

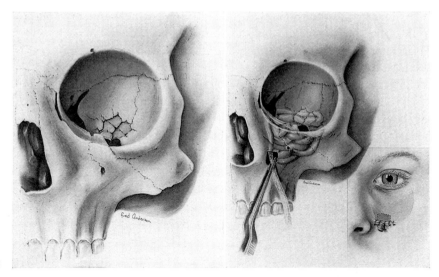

a   b

Fig.5. A Orbital floor 'blow-out' fracture. *B* Repair of orbital floor 'blow-out'
fracture by maxillary antrostomy and packing.

injury to the globe. In order to determine whether impairment of ocular
motility is the result of entrapment or motor nerve injury, the forced duction
test must be performed. This is accomplished by anesthetizing the conjunc-
tiva with a topical anesthetic agent and then grasping the muscular attachment at the deepest point in the mid-portion of the inferior conjunctival
sulcus. Inability to rotate the globe upward with gentle traction indicates
that the inferior rectus muscle is trapped in the fracture line.

Roentgenographic studies may show an opacification of the entire maxillary antrum on the involved side or a density in the superior portion of the
antrum. Polytomography will frequently show specific bone fragments and
spicules depressed into the antrum.

The most common location of this fracture is shown in figure 5 A. Since
the injury usually occurs in older children and the problem of unerupted
dentition is seldom an issue, treatment can usually be accomplished satisfactorily by approaching the antrum through the anterior wall of the maxilla
as shown in figure 5 B. The fragments are reduced to a normal anatomic
position, with care being taken to avoid over-reduction. The forced duction

test is repeated to determine that the reduction has not resulted in entrapment of the inferior rectus, and the antrum is packed with ½-inch selvage gauze impregnated with Vaseline® and an antibiotic ointment. In order to assure adequate sinus drainage, a nasoantral window is created, and the packing is most conveniently brought out through the Caldwell-Luc incision.

In those few cases where this treatment is inadequate, it may be necessary to explore the floor of the antrum. A reconstructive implant of cartilage, bone from the anterior maxillary wall, Supramid®, or Silastic® may be employed to restore orbital floor strength and contour. Since extrusion is one of the complications associated with the implantation of alloplastic materials, this should be avoided unless absolutely necessary.

Because of the risk of associated ocular injuries and postoperative complications pertaining to ocular motility, consultation with an ophthalmologist should be routine.

Mandibular Fractures

Fractures of the mandible are much less common in children than in adults because of the relative strength and elasticity of this bone during the younger years. In our experience, they account for approximately 4 % of the total number of mandibular fractures seen in a general acute and referral hospital center. Most of these fractures will involve the condylar neck, but approximately one third will involve the body or symphysis of the mandible. The issues related to growth, deciduous dentition, and unerupted teeth make the management of these fractures a specialized problem, and dental consultation is extremely important.

Common findings are malocclusion, deviation of the mandible with opening, pain near the fracture line, step-off deformity in the region of the fracture, crepitus, and false motion.

Roentgenographic studies are important in documenting the exact nature and location of the fractures. The panoramic X-ray view is quite helpful in many instances.

Fractures of the mandibular body will usually occur through the tooth buds of unerupted teeth in younger children. Whenever possible, it is best to avoid open reduction and direct interosseous wiring. In some instances, inability to obtain satisfactory reduction or instability after this has been obtained will necessitate an open approach. An example of this type of fracture is shown in figures 6 A, B, and C. Note that in figure 6 B, the drill holes

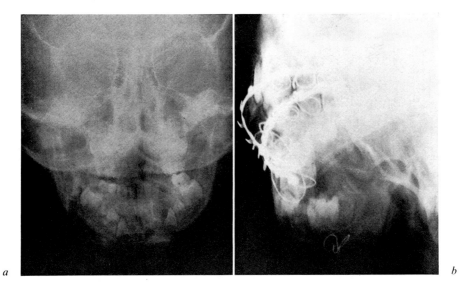

a   b

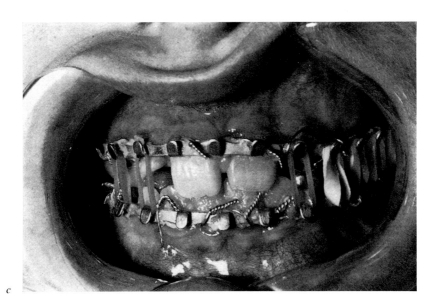

c

Fig.6. A Bilateral mandibular fracture in a 5-year-old child. B X-Rays showing the repair by means of direct interosseous wiring, arch bars, and elastic bands. C Oral view showing the immobilization appliance. Note the visible perimandibular supporting wire.

for the interosseous wiring have been made very close to the inferior margin of the mandible to avoid passing through the tooth bud. The wiring is accomplished with 26 gauge stainless steel wire in a figure-eight fashion. When the arch bars must be ligated to deciduous teeth, it is particularly important to support the arch bar with several circumferential wires around the mandible in order to avoid avulsion of these teeth. In figure 6C, one of the circumferential wires can be seen.

Because of their instability, fractures involving the mental symphysis almost always require open reduction and direct interosseous wiring in addition to the application of arch bars. The second important factor in this problem is that the blood supply essential for healing is least adequate in the region of the mental symphysis.

Historically, management of condylar neck fractures in children has been a controversial area. There have been three schools of thought regarding treatment: (1) open surgical reduction with direct interosseous wiring; (2) conservative management employing intermaxillary fixation or mandibular splints, and (3) no treatment.

Some authors have felt that the treatment options and management-outcome were closely related to the severity of the condylar neck fracture in the young patient. One classification system treated the fracture as minimal when there was good occlusion and no deviation of the chin on opening but moderate to severe if there was premature molar contact (interceptive malocclusion), deviation of the chin to the side of the fracture on opening, and loss of chin protrusion. Other observers have noted that there is no relationship between eventual outcome and the severity of the fracture unless the condylar head is so severely displaced (external auditory canal or other remote location) that it cannot conceivably realign itself and develop contact with the more distal portion of the mandible. It has been noted that in most instances the mandibular condyle displaces medially, anteriorly, and inferiorly.

The complications that have been seen in association with condylar neck fractures are malocclusion ('open bite' deformity), ankylosis or limited motion of the temporomandibular joint, pain on function, pseudoarthrosis, arthritis, and growth disorders.

DESSNER [5] was one of the first authors to provide careful documentation of favorable outcome with no treatment. He showed complete anatomic healing with remodeling of the dislocated condyles. There was no evidence of malocclusion or temporomandibular joint problems in his patient series.

These observations were confirmed in the experimental laboratory by

WALKER [9] and BOYNE [2]. WALKER [9] performed osteotomies and dislocated the condyle in nine rhesus monkeys. Comparing this procedure with direct interosseous wiring and no treatment, he observed that all animals had a useful TM joint articulation, an upright condyle, normal occlusion, and normal ramus height. BOYNE [2] did a similar study comparing open reduction and interosseous wiring with intermaxillary fixation for 3 weeks. There was a control group that received no treatment. He demonstrated that there was no condyle resorption and a complete recontouring and healing in all animals.

More recent clinical observations have included those of COOK and MACFARLANE [4] who observed bony union in all their patients and normal anatomical relationships in most. There was not correlation between fracture severity and the eventual outcome. They also demonstrated that early function did not produce a false joint at the fracture line. In 1971, LEAKE et al. [6] provided long-term roentgenographic studies that: (1) showed gradual realignment of the condylar head in spite of severe dislocation, and (2) the condylar neck growth center remains active after fracture.

On the basis of these reports and others, there appears to be strong evidence in support of a conservative approach to the management of children who sustain condylar neck fractures. Historically, the initial movement was from open reduction to intermaxillary fixation and the use of dental splints designed to prevent the 'open bite' deformity. Subsequently, the movement has been toward no treatment at all, except when there are other associated mandibular fractures or extreme instances of condylar head dislocation.

Summary

This chapter has emphasized the relative infrequency of severe skeletal maxillofacial injuries in children. When they do occur, it is extremely important that they be approached by a team of physicians, each of whom is competent to manage the injury and complications related to his specialty. Particular attention must be given to the issues of general facial bone growth as well as future dental development. All operative procedures must be designed to avoid further injury to unerupted teeth, and the traditional methods of immobilization must be modified in order to avoid the avulsion of deciduous teeth.

References

1 BORGES, A. F.: Elective incisions and scar revision (Little, Brown, Boston 1973).
2 BOYNE, P.J.: Osseous repair and mandibular growth after subcondylar fractures. J. oral. Surg. 25: 300–309 (1967).
3 CONVERSE, J.M. and SMITH, B.: Enophthalmos and diplopia in fractures of the orbital floor. Br. J. plast. Surg. 9: 265 (1957).
4 COOK, R.M. and MACFARLANE, W.I.: Subcondylar fracture of the mandible: a clinical and radiographic review. Oral Surg. 27: 297–304 (1969).
5 DESSNER, L. and HOLM, O.F.: Fracture dislocations of the mandibular condyle in children. Nord. Med. 59: 96 (1958).
6 LEAKE, D.; DOYKOS, J.; HABAL, M.B., and MURRAY, J.E.: Long-term follow-up of fractures of the mandibular condyle in children. Plast. reconstr. Surg. 47: 127–131 (1971).
7 FORT, R. LE: Fractures de la mâchoire supérieure. Congr. int. de méd., sect. de chir. gen., Paris 1900, pp. 275–278.
8 National Safety Council: Accident facts (National Safety Council, Chicago 1975).
9 WALKER, R.V.: Traumatic mandibular condylar fracture dislocations: effect on growth in the macaca rhesus monkey. Am. J. Surg. 100: 850–863, 1960.
10 WEBSTER, R.C.; DAVIDSON, T.M., and SMITH, R.C.: Practical suggestions on facial plastic surgery – how I do it. Laryngoscope 86: 1280–1284 (1976).

BYRON J. BAILEY, MD, Wiess Professor and Chairman, The Department of Otolaryngology, The University of Texas Medical Branch, *Galveston, TX 77550* (USA)

Adv. Oto-Rhino-Laryng., vol. 23, pp. 169–191 (Karger, Basel 1978)

Neurovestibular Examination of Infants and Children[1]

LYDIA EVIATAR and ABRAHAM EVIATAR

Department of Pediatrics (Neurology), The Bronx Lebanon Hospital Center, and
Department of Otorhinolaryngology, A. Einstein College of Medicine, Bronx, N.Y.

Introduction

Vestibular dysfunction in adults may be manifested by attacks of vertigo, unsteadiness, and rarely loss of postural control. Similar symptoms may occur in children; however, loss of postural control occurs more frequently in children than in adults. Of additional concern in pediatrics is the distinction between symptoms from an immature vestibular system versus vestibular dysfunction. Abnormals responses in children need further clarification to distinguish whether the problem rests primarily with the vestibular apparatus *per se*, vestibular pathways, or with abnormalities in the visual, motor or proprioceptive systems which jointly contribute to the acquisition of motor milestones.

It is particularly important, in deaf children, that vestibular function be evaluated since both the labyrinth and cochlea are in close anatomical relationship and may be affected by the same noxious or developmental factors. Children with congenital deafness occasionally present with delay in acquisition of postural control and, if tested appropriately, abnormal vestibular function may be demonstrated.

Methods of Evaluation

Methods of evaluation have evolved from myriads of observations by embryologists, anatomists, physiologists and clinicians over the years.

[1] This work is supported in part by Research Grant Number NS-10238-01, from the National Institute of Neurological Diseases and Blindness.

The development of the vestibular organ (membranous labyrinth) occurs early in embryonal life and is completed in the 30-mm embryo [4]. The maturing ampullary cristae become active as early as the eighth or ninth week of fetal life and a feeble Moro reflex (from vestibular receptors) can be elicited as early as the ninth to tenth week of gestation [12]. Brainstem reflexes that control eyeball movements begin to operate by the twelfth week of gestation and become fully established by the 24th week [1, 5, 13]. The vestibular nerve is the first to myelinate among central nervous system tracts, this occurring around 16 weeks of intrauterine life, at about the same time as myelination of the intersegmental tract systems of the cervical spinal cord [11].

Vestibular receptor systems in the internal ear become reflexogenically fully active by the 32nd week, at which time a fully developed Moro reflex can be elicited [15]. These observations suggest that vestibular afferents are mature and functional in early stages of human development. The acquisition of body equilibrium depends on proprioceptive and visual, as well as vestibular input, for information. The correction of body position relative to the various changes in space depends on the ability of the muscles and the whole motor system to respond to the proper stimulus in a coordinated fashion. Since widespread connections in the central nervous system are involved, precise localizazion of a lesion or the explanation for failure of an appropriate response to a specific stimulus is difficult. An abnormal response may be due to inability of the sensory systems to receive information (visual, vestibular or proprioceptive disturbances), to inability of cortical centers to process the information, or to damage of the motor systems (pyramidal or extrapyramidal) which prevents normal performance.

In order to understand the role of the vestibular system in the development of equilibrium, a review of its anatomy is appropriate [10].

The peripheral endings of the vestibular portion of the eighth nerve are on the hair cells of the maculae of the utricle and saccule and on the hair cells of the cristae in the ampullae of the semicircular canals. While the semicircular canals respond to angular movements, the utricles and saccules are concerned mainly with gravitational motion and linear acceleration. The peripheral nerve endings collect impulses transmitted by the hair cells of the maculae and cristae as a result of motion of the endolymphatic fluid. These afferent impulses are transmitted to the bipolar cells of the vestibular ganglion. The axons of the bipolar cells of the vestibular ganglion pass through the internal auditory canal and reach the medulla alongside the cochlear nerve. Most of the fibers end in the four vestibular nuclei clustered in the lateral part of the floor of the fourth ventricle. A few fibers pass directly from the nuclei to the cerebellum, ending in the cortex of the flocculo-nodular lobe. The fastigio bulbar tract arises from the cerebellum. Its fibers terminate in the vestibular nuclei and on the hair cells of the labyrinth. An additional efferent component arises in the lateral vestibular nucleus and terminates on the vestibular hair cells, exerting central influence on the receptors of the membranous labyrinth.

Two vestibulospinal tracts derive from the vestibular nuclei. The lateral tract (uncrossed) comes from the lateral vestibular nucleus and extends to the sacral level of the cord. The medial tract, with both crossed and uncrossed fibers, comes chiefly from the medial and spinal vestibular nuclei and extends through the cervical level of the cord, ending in lower motor neurons in the anterior horn of the cervical cord. Impulses descending in these tracts assist the local myotatic reflexes and reinforce the tonus of the extensor muscles of the head and neck and of the limbs, producing enough extra force to support the body against gravity and maintain an upright posture.

Fibers from the vestibular nuclei are carried rostrally in the medial longitudinal fasciculus and constitute the vestibulomesencephalic tract, which is distributed to the nuclei of the cranial nerves supplying the ocular muscles. Vestibular and optic reflexes permit us to keep the eyes fixed on stationary objects while the head and body are in motion. Movement of the head to the right, for instance, causes a small flow of endolymph in the horizontal semicircular canals directed to the left – due to fluid inertia, which makes it lag behind the movement of the head. Vestibular impulses, sent to the abducens and oculomotor nuclei, induce slow eye deviation to the left in order to keep the fields of vision unchanged. As they reach maximal deviation, the eyes quickly jerk back to the mid position. Persistent stimulation of hair cells in the appropriate ampullae of the semi-circular canals produces vestibular impulses which induce slow deviation of the eyes toward the direction of the endolymphatic current. This continues until the ocular muscles reach their maximum tension, at which point the eyes quickly return to their resting position. When these eye movements occur in sufficiently rapid succession to resemble oscillations, they are referred to as 'nystagmus'. The direction of nystagmus is designated in accordance with the direction of the fast component. This component is dependent on the integrity of the vestibular nuclei.

Recording of the oculomotor responses to peripheral labyrinthine stimulation by rotation or caloric stimulation has been widely used as a

Table I. Neurovestibular examination: 0–4 years

Extraocular motion (3, 4, 6 cranial nerves)
  Strabismus?
  Spontaneous nystagmus?
Following objects:
  Wandering gaze   >   2 weeks
  To midline   > 4–6 weeks
  For 180°   >   6 weeks
Fundoscopy
Refraction (direct or indirect)
Cranial nerves 2, 5, 7–12
Posture-tone:

Head control   { prone
Body control   { supine
              { sitting
              { standing

Gait with eyes open and blindfolded
Deep tendon reflexes
Developmental reflexes
Visual-motor coordination
  Finger-light pursuit
  Building with blocks
  Copying figures
Audiometry adapted to patient's age
Electronystagmography
  Position test
  Torsion swing
  Ice-cold caloric
  Optokinetic > 6 months

Table II. Neurovestibular examination: 4 years to adult

Coordination tests	Vibration sense
Heel-toe gait	Stereognosis
Finger-nose	Two-point discrimination
Heel-shin	
Diadochokinesis	Romberg
Position in space: fingers	Stepping test
(kinesthetic sense): limbs	
	Gait (blindfolded)
Equilibrium reactions	Audiometry
	Electronystagmography (full test)

Table III. Group I: 0–4 months

Primitive reflexes (vestibular and proprioceptive afferents)
    Neck righting (fig. 1)
    Asymmetric tonic neck (fig. 2)
    Symmetric tonic neck
    Moro (fig. 3)
Vestibular tests
    Vertical acceleration (fig. 4)
    Doll's eye phenomenon (fig. 5)

Table IV. Six to 48 months

Vestibular righting responses (patient blindfolded)
    Head over body righting > 24 months
Head righting
    Prone (fig. 6)
    Supine (fig. 7)
    Sideways (fig. 8)
Buttress (fig. 9)   > 24 months
Hopping (fig. 10) > 24 months
Parachute (fig. 11)

method for investigating the integrity of the vestibular system. However, complete examination of the vestibular system also includes assessment of its role in maintenance of tone and postural control through the vestibulospinal tract and the central connections with the reticular formation, basal ganglia, and posterior superior temporal gyrus. Integration of vestibular and motor responses occurs in the red nucleus. Extensive experimental evidence suggests that the red nucleus controls righting responses in animal and man. Indeed, animal studies of cortical transection below the level of the red nucleus demonstrate total inability to right the head or body [16].

Righting reflexes appear at about 6 months of age and usually persist throughout life in humans. They constitute an important developmental motor milestone toward the acquisition of spatial orienting mechanisms. Since optical and vestibular righting reflexes are similar, evaluation of the vestibular responses is performed with the child blindfolded.

The cortical representation of the vestibular system is at the level of the posterior superior gyrus of the temporal cortex. Experimental evidence

Table V. Electronystagmography

Positional
  Prone
  Supine
  Right lateral
  Left lateral
  Sitting – head right
  Sitting – head left
Perrotatory
  Torsion swing
  (with 10r/60″)
Calculation
  Number of beats left
  Dif. $> 25\%$ ⇥ dir. prep.
  Amplitude
  Frequency
  Duration (post-rotation)
Cold caloric irrigation
Bithermal caloric irrigation > 4 years
Optokinetic nystagmus > 6 months
  Film strip at 3°/sec
  Film strip at 16°/sec

---

suggests that inhibitory and facilitatory reflexes are transmitted from the temporal cortex to the lower vestibular centers [2]. Paroxysmal discharges originating in this area would be responsible for occurrence of vestibular seizures.

The following enumerates the various tests and examinations:

(1) The neurovestibular examination is divided into 2 parts: (a) a general neurological examination preceded by a detailed perinatal and postnatal history (tables I, II), and (b) specific neurovestibular testing adapted to the patient's age, including postural reactions (tables III, IV) and electronystagmography (table V).

(2) Ear, nose and throat examination ro rule out malformations connected directly or indirectly with dysfunction of the equilibrium system.

(3) Skull X-rays with views of the internal auditory canals.

(4) Hearing test, adapted to the patient's age.

(5) Blood studies, including fasting blood sugar, BUN, Ca, phosphate, alkaline phosphotase, electrolytes, T_3 and T_4, routine urinalysis, and amino

acid chromatography of urine to rule out metabolic abnormalities which contribute to imbalance, vertigo or delayed acquisition of postural control.

(6) Electroencephalography when indicated, especially in children with vertigo and attacks of loss of postural control in whom seizures should be excluded.

General Neurological Examination

The neurological examination is adapted to the patient's age and degree of central nervous system (CNS) maturation and should evaluate, especially, those parts of the CNS whose function is intimately related to the vestibular system, principally the visual proprioceptive and motor systems. Testing for vision, ocular alignment and ability to follow can be performed in the very young infant and will provide information about cranial nerves 3, 4, and 6 (table I). Direct or indirect ophthalmoscopy can also be performed. Presence or absence of corneal and gag reflexes, facial asymmetry with muscular activity, and abnormal tongue motions may be easily ascertained. The rooting reflex helps to bring out a full range of tongue motions in the neonate. Evaluation of muscle tone and of postural reactions is important, since both are dependent on vestibulospinal reflexes which reinforce myotatic reflexes in the extensor muscles of the limbs. Since head control is dependent on visual cues as well as on proprioceptive and vestibular functions, it should be tested in the blindfolded child to eliminate visual input. Tests for visual motor coordination provide information about integration of visual, cerebellar, pyramidal and extrapyramidal pathways and can be performed at early ages by such maneuvers as finger-light pursuit in the 6-month-old, dexterity in block building around 1 year of age, and ability to copy figures at 3 years.

Audiometry is also adapted to age level. An infant screener is used in the very young. Blink, cry, and autonomic responses may be used in the infant and, when no responses are obtained, one may resort to auditory evoked responses. By 4 or 5 months of age, orientation to sound occurs. By the age of 2 years, play audiometry is fairly reliable.

Beyond age 4 years, most of the same neurological test procedures that are used in adults may be used in children (table II). Elaborate coordination tests are possible in a child whose confidence and cooperation are gained. Rapid alternate motions, which provide information on cerevellar and basal ganglia function, can be performed. Proprioceptive input is assessed from the ability of the subject to locate his limbs in space, the Romberg test, and from the gait while blindfolded. Children beyond 4 years of age may also be required to mark time in place with eyes closed at the intersection of two perpendicular lines (stepping test). With vestibular disease, the patient cannot retain the initial starting position but rather sways laterally with a significant deviation, often of greater than 45°.

Sensory modalities, including stereognosis, two-point discrimination, and vibration should be tested.

Postural reactions. For simplicity of presentation, we divide the children into four groups according to age and level of maturation of the central nervous system.

Group I: 0–4 Months (table III)

As already mentioned, the pyramidal tract and the medial lemniscus are not yet myelinated. Postural patterns are very primitive and controlled at the brainstem level.

The tonic neck reflexes, elicited by passive or active motions of the head relative to fixed position of the body, are most characteristic od this age group. Head movements elicit impulses derived from the semicircular canals as well as proprioceptive stimuli from the cervical vertebrae and muscles. Normal responses depend on the integrity of the vestibular and proprioceptive impulses and on the efferent motor pathways. A well-coordinated reflex does not separate the components but indicates a normal overall integrated response.

Neck righting (fig. 1). Forceful rotation of the head from the midline to one side, in an infant lying supine, produces a righting reaction of the whole body which rotates to the same side as the head.

Asymmetric tonic neck reflex (ATN) (fig. 2). The baby lies supine with his head in the midline position. The examiner forcefully rotates the head to one side while restraining the infant's chest to prevent neck-righting. The expected response includes flexion of the extremities on the side of the occiput and extension of limbs on the side of the face.

Symmetric tonic neck reflex (STN). The baby is held in the horizontal prone position with the examiner's hand under the chest. Dorsiflexion of the head elicits extension of the upper extremities and flexion of the lower ex-

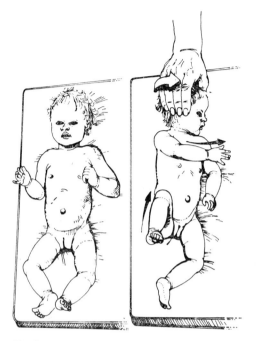

Fig. 1.

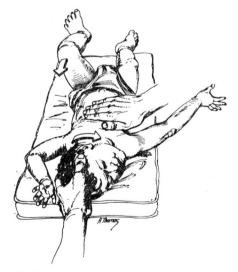

Fig. 2.

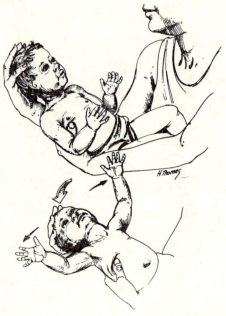

Fig. 3.

tremities. Ventroflexion elicits flexion of upper extremities and extension of lower extremities.

Moro reflex (fig. 3). The baby lies supine with head ventroflexed and is supported by the examiner's hand. The reflex is elicited by permitting the head to drop backward about 30° in relation to the trunk. The normal response is an extension and abduction of the arms followed by an embrace.

When the response is inadequate, it may be the result of a vestibular abnormality or an abnormality of the proprioceptive or motor systems. This may be demonstrated by performing additional specific neurological testing for each system separately.

Specific vestibular reflexes are vertical acceleration and Doll's eye phenomenon.

Vertical acceleration (introduced by the authors) (fig. 4). The baby is held in supine position, on the examiner's extended forearms. The head and trunk are aligned parallel to the ground. Rapid downward acceleration is produced to the baby's horizontal body by the examiner who bends his

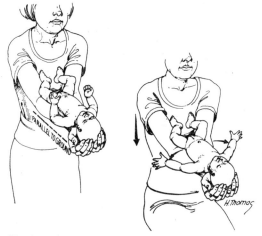

Fig. 4.

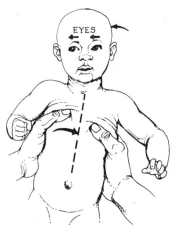

Fig. 5.

knees. The appropriate response for the baby is slight dorsiflexion of the head and abduction and extension of the arms with fanning of the hands. The response is similar to the Moro reflex. However, the absence of head motion in this instance eliminates proprioceptive input from the cervical vertebrae, while the vertical acceleration provides vestibular impulses to the utricle and saccule.

Doll's eye phenomenon (fig. 5). Another type of vestibular stimulation is provided by rotation. The baby is held vertically and facing the examiner, with the examiner's hands surrounding the baby's trunk. The baby's head is bent forward 30° over the body.

Rotation of the baby around the examiner's axis produces deviation of the eyes and head opposite to the direction of rotation. This reflex, called the Doll's eye phenomenon, usually persists for the first 2 weeks of life in the normal, full-term neonate and up to 6 weeks of age in the full-term baby, born small-for-gestational age. It may persist for three months in the premature [8]. When vestibular responses mature, most likely as a result of better integration at the level of the vestibular nuclei, the Doll's eye phenomenon is substituted by nystagmus with the quick component in the direction of rotation. This response can be recorded with electronystagmography.

Group II: 4–6 Months

This is an intermediate group from the developmental standpoint. Some babies will still have primitive tonic neck reflexes while others will show a higher level of maturation and some righting reflexes will be elicited. Both extremes will represent the normal range of development at this age and absence of righting responses is not considered pathological. Electronystagmography will be helpful in recording responses to perrotatory stimulation and if this response is absent, ice-cold caloric (ICC) irrigation can be performed and will provide additional information about each individual labyrinth.

Group III: 6–18 Months

Dendritic synapses between cortical neurons and myelination of the pyramidal track and medial lemniscus are far advanced in this age group.

Integration of visual, proprioceptive, and vestibular stimuli occurs at the level of the red nucleus, resulting in more elaborate motor responses called 'righting reflexes'.

The righting reflexes are elicited by tilting the patient abruptly and changing his center of gravity. The acceleration imposed on the vestibular apparatus elicits stimuli which bring upon righting of the head and protective reactions of the extremities.

As mentioned previously, vestibular righting reflexes are checked in the blindfolded individual in order to eliminate optical righting reflexes which are analogous responses but from different afferent stimuli.

The most characteristic reflexes to be examined in this group are the *head righting reflexes* obtained by changing the patient's position rapidly from upright to prone or supine or by tilting him sideways.

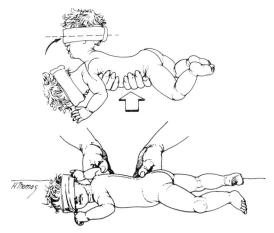

Fig. 6.

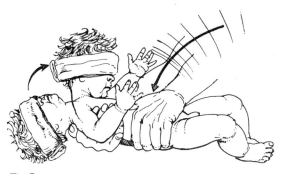

Fig. 7.

In each testing situation, the change of position in space elicits vestibular responses which induce head righting whereby the mouth and eyes become horizontal to the ground (fig. 6–8). Another example of head righting is the 'buttress' or 'propping reaction' (fig. 9). This reflex is tested in the sitting position. The examiner holds the baby around the chest tilting him sideways and forward. The normal response is a propping reaction of the upper extremities with righting of the head. Acquisition of this reflex enables the child to maintain his equilibrium in sitting.

Additional reflexes in which labyrinthine stimulation contributes to a total body response are:

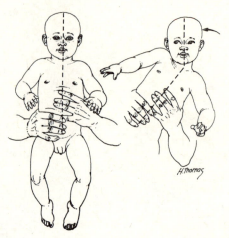

Fig. 8.

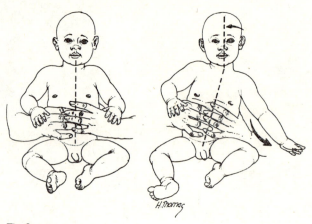

Fig. 9.

Body righting over head. This reflex is similar to the primitive neck righting of the infant in which turning of the head sideways induces turning of the body in the same direction. In the older child, the rolling over occurs in a segmental fashion gradually involving the shoulder girdle, the trunk, and the lower extremities. In most instances, this is followed by standing on all fours and crawling. In the 8-month-old, this maneuver can lead to voluntary sitting. These righting responses are the basic mechanisms by which the child acquires motor milestones such as rolling over, crawling, and sitting.

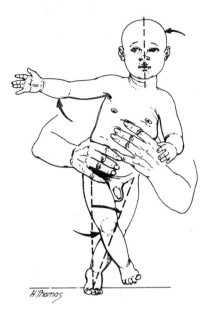

Fig. 10.

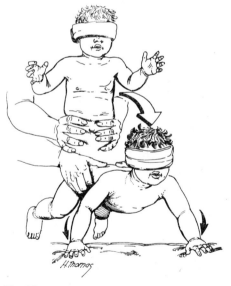

Fig. 11.

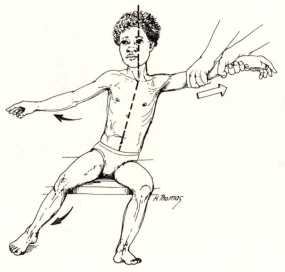

Fig. 12.

Hopping reaction (fig. 10). This reflex is present in the child who has already acquired standing balance. The baby is tested in the standing position. The examiner holds him around the chest and applies a gentle tilt sideways, foreward, and backward. A positive reflex is the initiation of a few steps in the direction of tilt, followed by righting of the head. This reflex constitutes the basis for acquisition of walking balance.

Parachute (fig. 11). This is also called the sentinel reaction since it is a basic protective body mechanism. Vertical downward acceleration is applied to the baby who is held around his chest. Immediate extension of arms with abduction and extension of fingers occurs as well as righting of the head.

Some righting reflexes persist throughout life (the parachute, for instance). Others may be voluntarily inhibited in the older child or will be integrated into more complete equilibrium reactions which appear by age 4 years.

Vestibular Tests: Ages 4 Years to Adult

Equilibrium reactions. By age 4 years most normal children are sufficiently mature and cooperative to be tested for the presence of equilibrium reactions in addition to the regular neurological tests described in table II.

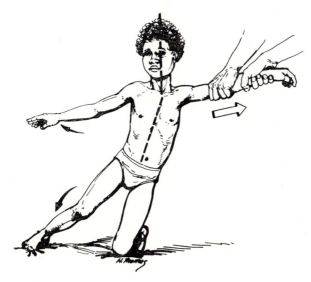

Fig. 13.

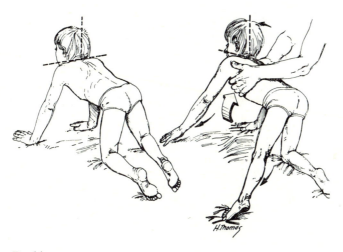

Fig. 14.

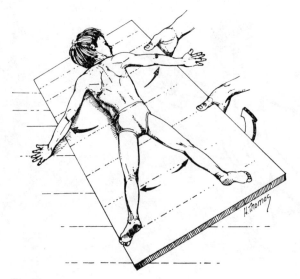

Fig. 15.

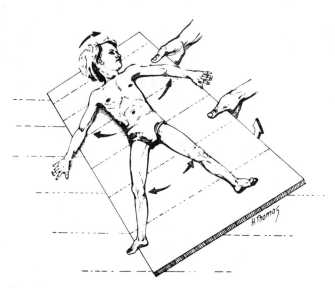

Fig. 16.

In the *sitting position* (fig. 12), the examiner pulls the child by his arm sideways. A normal reaction consists in 'righting' of the head and extension with abduction of the extremities on the side opposite the direction of tilt. Similar responses can be obtained in the *kneeling position* (fig. 13) or in the *four points kneeling* (fig. 14).

Additional whole body postural reactions can be elicited using a small *tilting board* on which the child lies either prone (fig. 15) or supine (fig. 16). The examiner tilts the board about 45° sideways and looks for the righting position of the head and the extension and abduction reactions of the extremities.

Equilibrium and postural reactions may be disturbed in neuromuscular disorders affecting the pyramidal or extrapyramidal pathways. They are significantly altered in diseases of the basal ganglia. In the absence of neuromuscular disorders, abnormal postural reactions may result from abnormal labyrinthine input.

Electronystagmography

Electronystagmography is a method of recording eye movements during positional testing and during labyrinthine stimulation by rotation and caloric irrigation. It is beyond the scope of this paper to discuss in detail this method which has been described in detail in many papers. Suffice it to say that for routine, clinical investigation and convenient office use, a one-channel AC dynograph recorder, the clinical type, is adequate. A positional test is first performed in the supine position, as well as in sitting, in the older child. The rotary stimulation is best provided, in our opinion, by the use of a torsion swing (several commercial types available on the market) which provides alternating angular acceleration of 180° to the right and left at a rate of 10 revolutions per 60 sec.

The test is done in a semi obscure room, with the baby blindfolded in order to eliminate ocular fixation and optokinetic nystagmus [6].

The stimulus provided by the torsion swing is sufficient to elicit oculomotor responses when they are present and provides the type of stimulation which closely mimics the physiological conditions encountered in daily situations. Young infants are seated in the mother's lap on the torsion swing. Her right hand maintains the baby's head flexed 30° over the body in order to align the lateral semicircular canals horizontal to the ground. Her left hand props the baby's trunk in the vertical position, close to her chest, so the axis of rotation is through the baby's trunk. The torsion swing is a non-threatening – even enjoyable – experience for the children who like to be rocked back and forth and, in most cases, cooperate well throughout the test. It is entirely different from the testing situation during a 360° rotation on the Barany chair which is non-physiological and may be frightening to children who become irritable and may have autonomic side effects such as pallor, nausea and vomiting. Recording of eye movements is done during stimulation with the torsion swing and after cessation of stimulus with the Barany method. In the majority of cases, the response ceases with cessation of perrotatory stimulation.

In the very young infant, a sinusoidal curve may be the only response obtained, signifying the conjugate eye movements in the direction opposite the direction of rotation (Doll's eye) over which will be slowly superimposed a few nystagmoid beats, changing direction with the direction of rotation. As the response fully matures (within 2–3 weeks in the full-term baby appropriate-for-gestational age, AGA), a good alternating nystagmus is obtained. The response thus recorded is the result of a summation of responses elicited from both labyrinths. Normally, the number of nystagmic beats in one direction equals the number of beats in the other direction. In cases where the number of beats in one direction exceeds by 25 % the number of beats in the opposite direction, a directional preponderance is suggested.

Additional testing with ICC irrigation of each ear canal for 10 sec may be performed in order to evaluate the response from each labyrinth individually.

The test is performed with the blindfolded baby in the supine position, his head ventroflexed 30°. Following a 10-sec irrigation with ice-cold water (temperature at the spout should be arouns 5 °C), the recording of oculomotor response is started. The direction of the nystagmus will be opposite the ear stimulated. As soon as a good response appears, the baby is turned to the prone position and the direction of nystagmus is reversed if the labyrinth is intact. As soon as this new response begins to fade, the baby is turned back to the supine position. The direction of nystagmus should then revert to the initial direction, away from the ear stimulated. In the majority of full-term babies, AGA, this response can be recorded with the first 3 or 4 weeks of life. It will be obtained later (within 6 weeks), in the full-term, small-for-gestational age and within 3 months in the premature. If the child is sleepy or very irritable during the test, the response may be inhibited or incomplete (response only in supine and prone, for instance). The test is performed in three positions with each irrigations in order to eliminate false responses, such as intensification of a latent nystagmus or a response from the other labyrinth. A full description of the method and its greater reliability over previously used methods appeared in a previous article [7]. 10 min should elapse before stimulating the other ear canal with ice-cold water. Absent response at the age when it should normally be present and under optimal testing conditions suggests an abnormal labyrinthine apparatus. Sleep or marked irritability may inhibit nystagmus and produce falsely abnormal results.

The ICC stimulation is a very crude method, testing for a response to a vigorous, non-physiological stimulus. It is thus used only in cases where serious doubts exist relative to the function of the vestibular apparatus, such as significant delay in head and postural control, abnormal responses to torsion swing, ingestion of ototoxic drugs or in the congenitally deaf child where abnormal vestibular function is suspected.

Slight differences in the quality of tracings have been found between the various age groups. A detailed statistical analysis of recordings obtained from 250 infants at various ages is the subject of a different paper. The general trend observed is towards a higher frequency of nystagmus, a higher amplitude of the beats, and a higher speed of the slow component with age in response to both perrotatory stimulation and ICC irrigation. A mature pattern is achieved around 18–24 months of age with very little variations thereafter. The duration of the nystagmic response to ICC stimulation seems to be a less accurate parameter of degree of maturation.

Optokinetic Nystagmus

Optokinetic nystagmus can be evaluated in most children starting between 3 and 6 months of age. Out of 19 children in this age group, 15 had good optokinetic responses to a rotating drum. As the children get older and pay more attention to the content of images they are seeing, better responses are obtained by projecting a rotating filmstrip. The nystagmus can be recorded in response to two speeds of rotation: 3 and 16°/sec, respectively. The frequency, amplitude of the maximal beat, and speed of slow component can be analyzed in response to the two rotation speeds. Abnormalities of tracings may be related to ocular problems, visual field deficits due to damage to optic tracts or optic radiations, to frontal or cerebellar lesions. The information obtained is extremely valuable in the evaluation of the overall neurovestibular picture. It is important to remember, however, that the pathways subserving optokinetic nystagmus are different from the pathways subserving vestibular nystagmus.

Bithermal Caloric Irrigation

Bithermal irrigation of external auditory meatus for 30 sec with 30 °C for cold and 44 °C for warm is used in children aged 4 years and above. A 10-min interval is allowed between two consecutive irrigations. The intensity of nystagmus represented by the speed of the slow component at culmination is used for calculation. Jongkee's formula $\pm 15\%$ was adopted for determination of labyrinthine preponderance; $\pm 18\%$ for directional preponderance [17]. This procedure lasts arouns 45 min and requires the child's cooperation and patience. It cannot, therefore, be used below age 4 years. The significance of directional and labyrinthine preponderance in children was discussed in a previous paper [9], and will be the subject of another paper in preparation by the authors.

Conclusion

An outline for a comprehensive neurovestibular evaluation of infants and children is presented. Children are divided into four groups according to age and level of central nervous system maturation, and the methods of testing take into account both levels of maturation and the influence of various systems on the acquisition of balance and postural control. Postural and equilibrium reactions serve as basic clinical parameters while electronystagmography is a useful laboratory tool.

References

1   BERGSTROM, L: Electrical parameters of the brain during ontogeny; in ROBINSON, Brain and early behaviour development in the fetus and infant. CASDS Study Group on Brain Mechanisms of Early Behaviour Development, pp. 15–37 (Academic Press, New York 1969).
2   CANTOR, F.K.: Vestibular-temporal lobe connections demonstrated by induced seizures. Neurology, Minneap. *21:* 507 (1971).
3   CRATTY, B.J.: Perceptual and motor development in infants and children (MacMillan, London 1970).

4 DEKABAN, A.: Neurology of early childhood (Williams & Wilkins, Baltimore 1970).

5 GESELL, A. and AMATRUDA, C.S.: The embryology of behavior: the beginning of the human mind (Harper, New York 1945).

6 EVIATAR, A.: The torsion swing as a vestibular test. Arch. Otolaryng., *92:* 437 (1970).

7 EVIATAR, A. and EVIATAR, L.: A critical look at the cold calorics. Archs Otolar. *99:* 361–365 (1974).

8 EVIATAR, L.; EVIATAR, A., and NARAY, I.: Maturation of neurovestibular responses in infants. Devl med. Child Neurol. *16:* 435–446 (1974).

9 EVIATAR, A. and WASSERTHEIL, S.: The clinical significance of directional preponderance concluded by electronystagmography. J.Lar.Otol. *85:* 355 (1971).

10 GATZ, A.J.: Manter's essentials of clinical neuroanatomy and neurophysiology (Davis, Philadelphia 1974).

11 HAMILTON, W.J. and MOSSMAN, H.W.: Human embryology: prenatal development of form and function; 4th ed. (Hoffer, Cambridge 1972).

12 HOLT, K.: Movement and Child Development. Clinics in Developmental Medicine, No.55 (Lippincott, Philadelphia 1975).

13 HOOKER, D.: The prenatal origin of behavior (University of Kansas Press, Lawrence 1952).

14 HUMPHREY, T.: Discussion; in ROBINSON Brain and early behaviour development in the fetus and infant. CASDS Study Group on Brain Mechanisms of Early Behavioural Development, pp.43–84 (Academic Press, New York 1969).

15 SCHULTE, F.J.; LINKE, I.; MICHAELIS, E., and NOLTE, R.: Excitation, inhibition and impulse conduction in spinal motoneurones of preterm, term and small-for-dates newborn infants; in ROBINSON Brain and early behaviour development in the fetus and infant. CASDS Study Group on Brain Mechanisms of Early Behavioural Development (Academic Press, New York 1969).

16 WALSHE, Review of Magnus and Rademaker 'Posture and Reflexes'. Brain *47:* 383 (1924).

17 YONGKEES, L.B.W. and PHILIPSZOEN, A.J.: Electronystagmography. Acta oto-lar. Suppl. *189* (1964).

Dr.L.EVIATAR, Department of Pediatrics (Neurology), The Bronx Lebanon Hospital Center, *Bronx, N.Y.* (USA)

Adv. Oto-Rhino-Laryng., vol. 23, pp. 192–205 (Karger, Basel 1978)

Genetic Counseling in Pediatric Otorhinolaryngology

David J. Harris and Basharat Jazbi

Genetic Counseling Center and Section of Otolaryngology,
The Children's Mercy Hospital, Kansas City, Mo.

All medical personnel who care for children must be aware of genetic factors in the etiology of the problems they see. In studies of admissions to pediatric services, approximately 25 % of the children have disorders that are either inherited or genetic factors contribute in the pathogenesis of the disease or malformations [8]. Although most otorhinolaryngologists collaborate with pediatricians in the care of children, at the present time experts in dysmorphology and other medical genetic entities are in tertiary care facilities and will probably remain there for economic reasons. The otorhinolaryngologist may be the one to suggest that a child needs further investigation. It is hoped that he will understand the geneticist's evaluation and recommendations and will be able to reinforce the latter. Consequently, the goal of this chapter is to point out those patients and families who would be candidates for genetic evaluation and counseling, its procedures, impact and possible continuing psychological needs of the family, rather than an exhaustive treatise or list of diseases.

The task of professionals in birth defects and genetic counseling today is both simpler and more difficult than it was before 1966. It is more difficult because there are more disorders to be aware of as well as an expanding literature of basic and applied science related to these disorders. It is simpler because of compilations and bibliographic tools that are now available. The landmark source is *Mendelian Inheritance in Man* by McKusick [21], which is a catalogue of inherited traits and diseases. *The Birth Defects Atlas and Compendium*, edited by Bergsma [2], and Smith's *Recognizable Patterns of Human Malformation* [30] are valuable resources to help establish a diagnosis. Finally, for problems in the head and neck area, Gorlin et al. [12] *Syndromes of the Head and Neck* is exhaustive.

Assessment of the Patient

Patients and families receiving genetic counseling are studied extensively before an opinion is given. A large segment of time is spent in obtaining an extended family history. Most physicians do not have the time to do this, but for both genetic and epidemiological reasons, when dealing with children, it is helpful to record accurately the data for the nuclear family. The least ambiguous method is to write down the names and birth dates of the parents and all of the children in the family. The dates and outcomes of all of the other pregnancies should also be noted. The parents should then be asked if anyone else is similarly affected. It has been assumed that the chief complaint and other pertinent historical information has been obtained.

It is essential for any child who has malformations of the head and neck to have a comprehensive examination so that anomalies of other organ systems can be recognized. With this information in hand, the clinician can use the various compendia to arrive at a diagnosis, and if he has the time and interest, provide appropriate counseling to the family. If the time and bibliographic resources are not available, it is better to refer the family to a center where the interest and expertise are available, rather than to give erroneous information and interpretation. Advances in reconstructive surgery of craniofacial malformations has stimulated the multidisciplinary approach to the care of these patients, involving representatives of general pediatrics, genetics, ophthalmology, otorhinolaryngology, neurosurgery, plastic surgery, radiology, psychiatry, anesthesiology, dentistry and orthodontics, social work, communications sciences, and nursing. Because so many disciplines are involved, a team approach is necessary to avoid fragmentation of care and omissions, particularly in the area of emotional support of both the patient and the family [22].

The detailed evaluation by a medical geneticist extends and completes the evaluation previously discussed. Much of the time whith the patient and the family will be devoted to obtaining the family history, although in some centers, a questionnaire completed by the family before being seen cuts down the amount of time required. (This may not be entirely advantageous, as the time spent obtaining the information is an opportunity for the building of rapport in addition to giving some hints regarding the psychological make-up of the concerned individuals, as well as familial psychosocial dynamics.) When working with pediatric patients, being able to interview both parents is helpful. Later on, when the flow of information is to the family, it is better not to burden one parent with the task of communicating what was said to the other.

For practical purposes, reliable information can usually be obtained for three generations: the child's generation, his parents', and grandparents'. In our center, family histories are obtained so that they can be processed by computer. This is done on worksheets with spaces for identification of the name of the proband (the person who presents for care), hospital number, family number, three diagnoses and their codes (either from the McKusick catalogue or the International Classification of Disease, Adapted), and a nuclear family consisting of the mother, father, and all pregnancies with dates of birth and death as well as clinical findings. Each kindred is composed of several nuclear family sheets which can be linked so that the computer can draw the pedigree [28]. Construction of a pedigree is an essential step in the diagnostic evaluation of a family that will receive genetic counseling, as it provides a graphic display of the family and the behavior of the disorder in that family.

The initial step of constructing a pedigree can be done by interview. It may require more than one sitting to obtain all of the birth dates, death dates and pregnancy losses. More distantly related individuals the parents do not know well may also have pertinent problems. Many families find that their relatives are initially unwilling to talk about problems, but that this may change. They may then be glad to release medical records or be seen themselves by the investigators.

It will be necessary, later on, to try to distinguish environmental from genetic factors. This is not always possible, but an attempt to identify factors in the pregnancy may be important. These include duration of marriage and interval between pregnancies, contraceptive usage, the number of menstrual cycles between discontinuation of oral progestational agents and conception, illnesses (particularly exanthematous febrile diseases or exposure to them), radiation and drugs including over-the-counter preparations and aspirin. Abnormal weight gain, the amount of amniotic fluid, and presenting fetal part may correlate with abnormalities [6]. The use of drugs in labor and delivery, the perinatal status of the infant and its developmental history may all need to be considered.

A few points about the physical examination are also worth mentioning. Some simple anthropometric measurements are helpful, particularly height, weight, and head circumference. Other external measurements, such as intercanthal and interpupillary distances are used in some centers [11]. An attempt should be made to describe abnormalities of visible structures. Ready recognition of some of them is admittedly subjective, however, it can become consistent. It is not a good idea to write pejorative comments such as 'FLK' in charts. Often, what appears to be an abnormality to an examiner is actually a familial characteristic in otherwise normal people, or may disappear in the first year of life. The remainder of the physical examination and routine urinalysis and blood count may give an indication of other affected organ systems. Specific laboratory studies may be necessary to complete the diagnosis, including radiographs, biochemical tests or chromosomal analysis. Because of the number of disorders now known to be genetic or in part genetically determined, even the experienced medical geneticist has to rely heavily on the library before arriving at a diagnosis and prediction of recurrence risks.

Genetic Principles

Prediction of the recurrence risk is a major part of the process of genetic counseling. It is by no means the only task that has to be accomplished. The fundamental rules are simple. One source of difficulty is *heterogeneity* which will be discussed later. The other source is the best interpretation of pedigree data. Sometimes this is straightforward. At other times, more advanced rules of probability have to be invoked in order to make correct inferences [23].

Hereditary information is stored in the sequences of bases of the DNA molecules that form a major portion of the chromosomes of all organisms. Although we now know relatively little about the control and mechanism of action of the hereditary elements, the *genes*, of higher organisms, this knowledge is not essential in understanding their behavior, which is essential for counseling. The particulate theory of inheritance antedated information about chromosomal behavior, however, it is easier to understand genetic inference by beginning with a description of chromosomal events. The somatic cells of man contain 46 chromosomes, which occur as 22 homologous *autosomes* and a pair of sex chromosomes: 2 X chromosomes in the female and an X and a Y in the male. These can be demonstrated in various tissues. Phytohemagglutinin transformed lymphocytes are the usual clinical source. The cells are arrested in *metaphase* and treated with a hypotonic medium to swell the chromosomes. After staining and photographing the metaphyses, the chromosomes in the photograph are arranged into a *karyotype*. During the last few years, techniques designated Q-banding, G-banding, and R-banding have allowed precise identification of human chromosomes, as well as demonstrated smaller rearrangements than were possible in the older, solid staining techniques [3]. What one sees is an already duplicated set of *diploid* chromosomes. In *mitosis*, replication precedes each division and the chromosomes separate so that there is no change in the number of chromosomes of each daughter cell. This is the normal process of cell division beginning with the zygote, however, both copying and separation (disjunction) errors can occur.

In *gametogenesis*, one replication precedes two divisions so that the ultimate result is a cell that is *haploid*, containing half the number of chromosomes of the somatic cells. The *prophase* (the stage of cell division in which the chromosomes become visible) is much more complicated. The homologous chromosomes associate, or *synapse*, and there are what appear to be overlaps or *chiasmata* which represent the exchange of material between members, or *crossing over*. Errors in disjunction may result in gametes that have extra or missing chromosomes. When fertilized with a normal gamete, the new zygote will be *trisomic* in the first instance and *monosomic* in the second. Theoretically, trisomy and monosomy for all chromosomes are possible, but in man many of them have reduced viability as shown by the incidence of such chromosomal abnormalities in first trimester aborted fetuses [7].

We will be able to understand the behavior of inherited traits from chromosomal behavior during meiosis. The location of a gene controlling a trait is its *locus*. The alternative states of a gene are called *alleles*. The appearance of an individual is its *phenotype*, while the underlying combination of two alleles, one for each chromosome of the pair which has the locus for that particular gene, is the individual's *genotype*. If both alleles are the same, the person is said to be a *homozygote;* if they are different, he is a *heterozygote*.

If one knows the genotypes of both parents, the genotypes of the offspring, as well as their frequency, can be predicted. If both parents are homozygous for the same allele, then all of their children will be the same: homozygous for the same allele. If one of the parents is a heterozygote, one half of the children will be heterozygotes and one half will be homozygotes, as shown in table I. The expected frequencies resulting from a mating of parents heterozygous for the same allele are shown in table II. Since the two offspring classes of heterozygotes are the same, their frequencies are summed, so that one half of the progeny of this mating are heterozygotes, one quarter are homozygotes for one allele, and one quarter are homozygotes for the other allele.

Table I. Offspring genotypes expected from a mating between a homozygous parent, AA, and a heterozygous parent, AA'

| | Gametes | Parental genotype AA' gametes | |
		A	A'
Parental genotype AA	A	½ AA	½ AA'

Table II. Offspring genotypes from a mating between two heterozygotes, each AA'

| | Gametes | Parental genotypes AA' gametes | |
		A	A'
Parental genotype AA'	A	½ AA	½ AA'
	A'	½ AA'	½ A'A'

Explicit identification of parental genotypes is not always possible. This is possible for some disorders that can be identified by biochemical techniques. For other traits, one has to make inferences from the appearance of the phenotype in the family. If the variant phenotype is present in the heterozygote for the unusual allele, that allele is said to be *dominant*. If an individual has to be homozygous for the trait to be demonstrable, that allele is said to be *recessive*. In studying human inheritance, adjustments have to be made for the small sample size and for sampling bias. For the clinician, however, certain simple rules are sufficient in most instances. For dominant traits, the sex ratio of affected persons is equal. There is an apparently vertical appearance of the trait in the pedigree, i.e. people in every generation are affected, and 50 % of the offspring or sibs of affected persons are affected. The mating type is that of a normal with an affected heterozygote as discussed above. In the case of recessive traits, the sex ratio is also equal, but the parents are normal. 25 % of the sibs are affected. The mating type corresponds to the last mating type previously discussed: two heterozygotes having a one in four risk for having abnormal offspring with each pregnancy. The parents of children with autosomal recessive traits are frequently consanguineous.

In addition to the pattern of inheritance observed for autosomal recessive traits, genes on the *X* chromosome follow a pattern that can be predicted from the behavior of the sex chromosomes. The normal female has two X chromosomes while the male has an X and a Y. Genes that are *X-linked* (located on the X chromosome) will behave like autosomal genes in the female, but will always be expressed in the male. A female who is carrying an X-linked recessive trait will appear normal. If she is mated with a normal male, half of her daughters will be carriers like herself, and half will be normal homozygotes. Half of her sons will be affected and half will be normal. If she has an X-linked dominant disorder, she will have the disease, as will half of her daughters as well as half of her sons.

There are complications that occur in human pedigrees. In families with an inherited disease, some of the members will have all of the clinical findings, while others may only have one or two. This is *variation in expressivity*. If a proportion of individuals who can be demontrated to have the appropriate genotype do not have any part of the phenotype, this is *variation in penetrance*. These definitions are used to explain skipping of generations in autosomal dominant traits as well as lack of affected persons in sibships. They are also used as a dodge in poorly understood disorders. Some of these effects may actually be due to modification by other genes.

Many common disorders, including cleft lip and palate are more complex. It is generally agreed that these phenotypes represent an interaction of several genetic and environmental factors. There are several terms used for this type of inheritance: *quantitative, multifactorial, polygenic* or *multilocal*. The basic theory was derived for study of continuous traits, such a stature, which can be shown to follow a normal distribution. Predictions of the values for offspring could then be made using properties of the variance and the mathematical analysis of the components of variation. The application of the mathematical principles of quantitative inheritance to discontinuous traits was made possible by the concepts of *liability* and *threshold* developed by FALCONER. Liability includes all of the factors that contribute to the likelihood of developing a disease or malformation. It is composed of environmental factors and several genetic loci whose alleles are generally additive in their effects. The liability can thus be arranged in a continuous, increasing scale. The point on the liability scale beyond which malformations or symptoms will appear is the threshold. The frequency of the trait in the general population and in relatives of the proband may be used to make predictions. The extensions made by EDWARDS allow the approximate recurrence risk to be estimated as the square root of the population frequency [5].

Counseling in this group of disorders is not entirely satisfactory. Many recommend the use of empirical risks derived from the population from which the family comes. Attempts are being made to use the mathematical theory of quantitative inheritance with more information obtained from the specific pedigree. What may ultimately be of greater importance is the demonstration of major genes defining risks [23].

Some Categories of Problems

There is a population of children that are born with head and neck problems who die either *in utero* or during the early neonatal period. Some have what appear to be isolated anomalies and some have recognizable syndromes. It is possible that this series of spontaneous and even induced abortions may account for the deviations from Mendelian expectations of traits that are thought to be genetic. Fetal wastage has been important in the epidemiology of chromosomal defects as previously mentioned. Consequently, fetal malformations, stillbirths and neonatal deaths must be evaluated. A careful physical examination should be done, photographs taken, good radiographs of the bones obtained, and if possible a thorough postmortem examination. This should include careful descriptions of malformations and weights of organs recorded. If malformations in several organ systems are observed, a piece of skin or gonad should be obtained under sterile conditions for establishment of a fibroblast culture which can be used for chromosomal analysis or biochemical studies [19]. This evaluation or that in the section on assessment will demonstrate which organ systems are involved and the literature can be searched for syndrome identification and appropriate samples sent to the proper laboratory.

The most common problems involving head and neck structures are cleft lip and palate (either isolated or combined) and hearing loss. The hearing loss may be either sensorineural or conductive. Several of the chromosomal disorders have facial clefts as well as other head malformations and hearing disorders. There are several disorders in which clefts are associated with other facial anomalies, such as lip pits, or skeletal dysplasia, such as the Kniest syndrome, which are clearly Mendelian traits [30]. Another important example is the Pierre Robin anomaly. This triad of micrognathia, cleft palate, and glossoptosis may appear as an isolated group of findings, as part of trisomy 18 or as the presenting features of the cerebro-costo-mandibular syndrome. The latter is an autosomal recessive, while the isolated mouth findings may be either sporadic or an autosomal dominant [4, 23, 29]. The majority of families in wich facial clefts appear do not have pedigrees that are consistent with simple, single locus inheritance. The familial incidence in several populations fits the expectations of multilocal inheritance, with decreasing risk as the dagree of relationship decreases, and increasing with the number of affected first degree relatives [1]. Attempts have been made to define parents at risk to give birth to children with facial clefts by an analysis of facial morphology, either externally or from X-rays, but the results have been ambiguous [17]. This has been used as an explanation for the ethnic variation in the incidence of facial clefting [27].

A large proportion of hearing loss is genetic in origin. There are a large number of rare syndromes which include deafness. Associations may be found between deafness and external ear malformations, integumentary system abnormalities, eye abnormalities, nervous system abnormalities, skeletal dysplasias, renal disorders, endocrine disease, cardiovascular disease, and lysosomal storage diseases and chromosomal anomalies. Genetic deafness may also be an isolated finding [16].

Each of several related diseases may have phenotypes that vary in severity and overlap one another. This is an exemple of *heterogeneity* which can make recognition of the etiology of deafness difficult. The deficiencies of lysosomal acid hydrolases are instructive. The prototype disorder is mucopolysaccharidosis I, or the Hurler syndrome. Most clinicians are familiar with the findings of short stature, frontal bossing, coarse features, corneal clouding, deafness, psychomotor retardation, hepatosplenomegaly, and the bone changes of dysostosis multiplex. The deafness is conductive in the Hurler syndrome, and both sensorineural or mixed deficits have been described in the other disorders of the group. The diagnosis used to be confirmed by the demonstration of increased dermatan sulfate and heparan sulfate in the urine. The tissues contain enlarged lysosomes which are composed of undegraded polymeric material. It is now known to be a deficiency of the enzyme iduronidase. A number of disorders with similar, but not identical phenotypes has been identified. At first, differentiation was partially done using pedigree and urinary biochemical findings. Now, enzymatic identification is possible in either plasma, white blood cells, or fibroblasts derived from skin biopsies or amniotic cell culture [20]. There are disorders that have clinical appearances similar to the Hurler syndrome that are not mucopolysaccharidoses. One of these is mannosidois. The original patients were severely affected in terms of facial appearance, short stature, sensorineural deafness and bone changes. They were shown to have abnormal lysosomes and to have decreased α-mannosidase which results in the accumulation of mannose-containing oligosaccharides that can appear in the urine [15, 26]. We are caring for a patient in whom the diagnosis was nearly missed because the facial features were nearly normal, and the X-rays had been initially read as normal. There may be many other patients like this, in whom the development of a simple, thin-layer chromatographic screening method may allow us to get a better idea of the incidence of this disorder, which may eventually be treatable [10, 13].

Proper family studies may help elucidate the pattern of inheritance of a disorder associated with a hearing deficit. The cervico-oculo-acoustic (Wildervanck) syndrome affects mainly girls [14]. They have a Klippel-Feil cervical fusion anomaly, an abducens paralysis and a Mondini type cochlear anomaly. It has been postulated that this is an X-linked dominant that is lethal in males. We have obtained an audiogram on the mother of such a child; there are mild losses at both the high and low frequencies. On the other hand, the father has a normal audiogram. We assume that this is consistent with the X-linked mode of inheritance that has been proposed for this disorder.

The largest group is composed of persons with isolated deafness without other recognizable features. All patterns of inheritance have been described. When families have been large enough, classical pedigrees have been constructed. There are families where parent to child transmission and the other criteria of dominant deafness have been evident, as well as sibships with multiple affected children and normal parents that satisfy criteria for recessive inheritance. Since deaf persons frequently marry deaf persons, the proportion of normally hearing offspring indicates that there are a number of recessive genes for deafness [9, 24]. Audiological evaluation of family members in addition to just obtaining subjective histories of deafness has allowed families to be classifiable into an inherited type [25, 32].

Otolaryngologists are rightly concerned about acquired conductive hearing loss from otitis media. Repeated middle ear infections may be a symptom of immunological deficiency states. There are heritable defects in all parts of the system, including immunoglobulins, cellular immunity, phagocytosis, and complement function. The immunology of some of the conditions is well understood. All genetic mechanisms are represented; however, there are still conditions in which the genetics is not clear. Increased problems with ear infections also may appear in allergic states, another disorder in which genetic factors are being shown to play an important role [31].

Another group of functions which can come to the otolaryngologist's attention are problems of swallowing and speech. Both of these may be the result of a central nervous system disease, either in the brain, cervical or

Table III. Genetic disorders in an ear, nose and throat clinic, excluding facial clefting

Type of disorder	Number of patients
Well-established genetic disorders	
Down's syndrome	1
Möbius syndrome	1
Charcot-Marie-Tooth disease	1
Congenital deafness	1
Possibly inherited disorders	
Cerebral giantism	1
Skeletal dysplasia (incompletely studied)	1
Multilocal disorders	
Congenital heart disease	3
Allergies	5
Hirschprung disease	1
Diabetes mellitus	1
Total	17

cranial nerve nuclei. Speech pathologists have been able to cluster speech patterns in a way that correlates with lesions at different levels of the nervous system. Many of the disorders are inherited and include entities such as hepatolenticular degeneration (Wilson's disease) and myotonic dystrophy[18].

Results of a Chart Survey of a Pediatric Ear, Nose and Throat Clinic

To demonstrate the prevalence of genetic disorders, it was felt that a sample of approximately 100 censecutive patients seen in the ear, nose and throat clinic of our hospital would demonstrate that the group of problems is relatively common, although the individual disorders are rare. 97 charts weres reviewed. Although most of the visits were related to acute or recurrent otitis media, there were 17 patients with underlying genetic disorders. The array is shown in table III. This series does not include cleft lip and palate, as these children are seen in a separate cleft palate clinic.

Genetic Counseling

Genetic counseling is a process in which the parents of an affected person or an affected person himself make a decision about future reproductive behavior and implement that decision. A number of steps have to be completed in order to carry this out. The pivotal concepts are of risk and of burden. The risk is the probability that the disorder will occur again. The burden is the effect that the disorder produces on the individual and his family. It is composed of many factors, including social and economic costs as well as handicap or other medical problems.

Risks cannot be estimated without the best possible diagnostic evaluation of the condition. It must be understood that in some cases, no diagnosis will be identified and that the diagnosis itself is really a probability statement. If a particular diagnosis seems to have a high enough probability of being a reasonable working hypothesis, the pedigree then has to be reexamined to establish the genetic diagnosis. Some family members may have to be examined. For a concrete example, as was pointed out earlier, the parents and siblings of deaf children ought to have audiograms in order to establish the behavior of the trait in the family. The extent of the calculations necessary for estimating the risk will then depend upon the trait and its behavior, as well as the information in the pedigree.

The next step is communication with the family. In addition to the quotation of the risks, there must be a discussion of the burden, with the counselor estimating what the components are likely to be, as well as listening to the family's reactions and feelings about the burden. The family may then be equipped to make a decision. Because it takes some time for a couple to react to and resolve the feelings generated by a severely affected child, this communication may be a slow process that takes months to complete. While this process is continuing and until the family definitely decides to have more children, it is essential that reliable contraceptive techniques are used to maintain the choices that are open.

Since people react differently to the same problem, some couples will elect not to risk having more children, while others will go ahead. In some instances, they will feel that the probability of having a normal child is high enough for them. At times, the varying decisions are based on a different perception of the burden. There are times when really no decision was made because the family denied that there was anything wrong. There is not much information on how well families implement their decisions, but a number of centers are trying to evaluate the outcome of their genetic counseling [23].

References

1 BEAR, J.C.: A genetic study of facial clefting in Northern England. Clin.Genet. *9:* 277 (1976).

2 BERGSMA, D. (ed.): Birth Defects Atlas and Compendium (Williams & Wilkins, Baltimore 1973).

3 BERGSMA, D. (ed.): Paris Conf. (1971), Supplement (1975): Standardization in human cytogenetics. Birth Defects: orig.art.ser. *9* (1975).

4 BIXLER, D. and CHRISTIAN, J.C.: Pierre Robin syndrome occurring in two related sibships. Birth Defects: orig.art.ser. *7:* 67 (1971).

5 BODMER, W.F. and CAVALLI-SFORZA, L.L.: Genetics, evolution and man (Freeman, San Francisco 1976).

6 BRAUN, F.H.; JONES, K.L., and SMITH, D.W.: Breech presentation as an indicator of fetal abnormality. J.Pediat. *86:* 419 (1975).

7 CARR, D.H.: Chromosomes and abortion; in HARRIS and HIRSCHHORN Adv.hum. Genet. *2:* 201 (1971).

8 CLOW, C.L.; FRASER, F.C.; LABERGE, C., and SCRIVER, C.R.: On the application of knowledge to the patient with genetic disease; in STEINBERG and BEARN Prog.med. Genet., vol.9, p.159 (Grune & Stratton, New York 1973).

9 CHUNG, C.S. and BROWN, K.S.: Family studies of early childhood deafness ascertained through the Clarke School for the Deaf. Am.J.hum.Genet. *22:* 630 (1970).

10 DESNICK, R.J.; THORPE, S.R., and FIDDLER, M.B.: Towards enzyme therapy for lysosomal storage diseases. Physiol.Rev. *56:* 57 (1976).

11 FEINGOLD, M. and BOSSERT, W.H.: Normal values for selected physical parameters: an aid to syndrome delineation. Birth Defects: orig.art.ser. *13* (1974).

12 GORLIN, R.J.; COHEN, M.M., jr., and PINDBORG, J.J.: Syndromes of the head and neck (McGraw Hill, New York 1975).

13 HUMBEL, R. and COLLART, M.: Oligosaccharides in urine of patients with glycoprotein storage diseases. I. Rapid detection by thin-layer chromatography. Clin. chim.Acta *60:* 143 (1975).

14 KIRKHAM, T.H.: Cervico-oculo-acusticus syndrome with pseudopapilloedema. Archs Dis.Childh. *44:* 504 (1969).

15 KJELLMAN, B.; GAMSTORP, J.; BRUN, A.; OCKERMAN, P., and PALMGREN, B.: Mannosidosis: a clinical and histopathological study. J.Pediat. *75:* 366 (1967).

16 KONIGSMARK, B.W. and GORLIN, R.J.: Genetic and metabolic deafness (Saunders, Philadelphia 1976).

17 KURISU, K.; NISWANDER, J.D.; JOHNSTON, M.C., and MAZAHERI, M.: Facial morphology as an indicator of genetic predisposition to cleft lip and palate. Am.J.hum. Genet. *26:* 702 (1974).

18 LAPOINTE, L.L.: Neurological abnormalities affecting speech; in TOWER The nervous system, vol.3, p.493 (Raven Press, Hewlett 1975).

19 MACHIN, G.A.: Chromosome abnormality and perinatal death. Lancet *i:* 549 (1974).

20 McKUSICK, V.A.: Heritable disorders of connective tissue; 4th ed., p.521 (Mosby, St.Louis 1972).

21 McKUSICK, V.A.: Mendelian inheritance in man (Johns Hopkins University Press, Baltimore 1975).

22 MUNRO, J.R.; Orbito-cranio-facial surgery: the team approach. Plastic reconstr. Surg. *55:* 170 (1975).

23 MURPHY, E.A. and CHASE, G.A.: Principles of genetic counseling (Year Book, Chicago 1975).

24 NANCE, W.E. and McCONNELL, F.E.: Status and prospects of research in hereditary deafness; in HARRIS and HIRSCHHORN Adv.hum.Genet., vol.4, p.173 (1973).

25 NORTHERN, J.L. and DOWNS, M.P.: Hearing in children (Williams & Wilkins, Baltimore 1974).

26 OCKERMAN, P.A.: A generalized storage disorder resembling Hurler's syndrome. Lancet *ii:* 239 (1967).

27 SAXEN, I.: Epidemiology of cleft lip and palate. An attempt to rule out chance correlations, Br.J.prev.soc.Med. *29:* 103 (1975).

28 SHOCKLEY, K. and HARRIS, D.J.: PDGRE: a computer program to graph human pedigrees. Am.J.hum.Genet. *28:* 88 (1976).

29 SCHIMKE, R.N.: The Pierre-Robin syndrome in sibs. Birth Defects: orig.art.ser. *2:* 222 (1969).

30 SMITH, D.W.: Recognizable patterns of human malformation; 2nd ed. (Saunders, Philadelphia 1976).

31 STIEHM, E.R. and FULGINITI, V.A.: Immunological disorders in infants and children, p.145 (Saunders, Philadelphia 1973).

32 TAYLOR, I.G.; HINE, W.D.; BRASIER, V.J.; CHIVERALLS, K., and MORRIS, T.: A study of the causes of hearing loss in a population of deaf children with special reference to genetic factors. J.Lar.Otol. *89:* 899 (1975).

D.J.HARRIS, MD, Chief, Associate Professor of Pediatrics, University of Missouri, Genetic Counseling Center, The Children's Mercy Hospital, *Kansas City, MO 64108* (USA)
B.JAZBI, MD, DLO, FAAP, Professor and Chief of Otorhinolaryngology, University of Missouri, School of Medicine, The Children's Mercy Hospital, *Kansas City, MO 64108* (USA)